ADDICTION AND THE VULNERABLE SELF

Modified Dynamic Group Therapy
for Substance Abusers

The Guilford Substance Abuse Series

EDITORS

HOWARD T. BLANE, Ph.D.

Research Institute on Alcoholism, Buffalo

THOMAS R. KOSTEN, M.D.

Yale University School of Medicine, New Haven

ADDICTION AND THE VULNERABLE SELF

Modified Dynamic Group Therapy for Substance Abusers

Edward J. Khantzian, M.D.
Kurt S. Halliday, M.A.
William E. McAuliffe, Ph.D.

Department of Psychiatry
Harvard Medical School
at The Cambridge Hospital
Cambridge, Massachusetts

THE GUILFORD PRESS
New York   London

© 1990 The Guilford Press
A Division of Guilford Publications, Inc.
72 Spring Street, New York, NY 10012

Printed in the United States of America

This book is printed on acid-free paper.

Last digit is print number: 9 8 7 6 5 4 3 2 1

Library of Congress Cataloging-in-Publication Data

Khantzian, Edward J.
    Addiction and the vulnerable self: modified dynamic group therapy for substance abusers (MDGT)/Edward J. Khantzian, Kurt S. Halliday, William E. McAuliffe.
        p. cm. — (The Guilford substance abuse series)
    Includes bibliographical references.
    Includes index.
    ISBN 0-89862-172-0
    1. Substance abuse—Treatment. 2. Self. 3. Psychodynamic psychotherapy. 4. Group psychotherapy. I. Halliday, Kurt S. II. McAuliffe, William E. III. Title. IV. Series.
    [DNLM: 1. Psychotherapy, Group. 2. Self Concept. 3. Substance Abuse—therapy. 4. Substance Dependence— therapy. WM 270 K45a]
    RC564.K53 1990
    616.86'0651—dc20
    DNLM/DLC
    for Library of Congress
                                                                    90-3821
                                                                    CIP

In order to preserve the confidentiality of persons who participated in the MDGT groups of the Harvard Cocaine Recovery Project, names and all other possible identifying information have been changed.

To our wives and children:

CarolAnn, Nancy Jo Modlish, and Susan, Jane, and John Khantzian

Carol, Susannah, and Katherine Halliday

Donna and Kaitlyn McAuliffe

ABOUT THE AUTHORS

The authors have many years' experience treating and conducting clinical research with addicts in a variety of clinical settings. **Edward J. Khantzian, M.D.** is Associate Professor in the Department of Psychiatry, Harvard Medical School at The Cambridge Hospital, where he is Principal Psychiatrist for Substance Abuse Disorders and Clinical Co-investigator of the Harvard Cocaine Recovery Project. Trained as a psychoanalyst, he is one of the founders of the Department of Psychiatry and was the first director of drug treatment programs for the hospital and the Cambridge-Somerville Mental Health Center. He is currently a staff psychiatrist at Danvers State Hospital, Danvers, Massachusetts.

Kurt Halliday, M.A. is Clinical Instructor in Psychology in the Department of Psychiatry, Harvard Medical School at The Cambridge Hospital. He is a research associate at the Harvard Cocaine Recovery Project, and was clinical director of Project Outreach, a NIDA-funded AIDS prevention and drug treatment program for intravenous drug users. Previously, he was the clinical consultant to Veritas Therapeutic Community in New York City. He was the first MDGT group leader in the Harvard Cocaine Recovery Project and is currently a doctoral candidate in clinical psychology at the New School for Social Research.

William E. McAuliffe, Ph.D. is Associate Professor in the Department of Psychiatry, Harvard Medical School at The Cambridge Hospital and Lecturer in the Department of Behavioral Sciences, Harvard School of Public Health. He is Director of Substance Abuse Research at The Cambridge Hospital. A clinical sociologist who received his doctorate in sociology from the Johns Hopkins University, he is Principal Investigator of both the Harvard Cocaine Recovery Project and Project Outreach. He is co-author of *Addict Aftercare: Recovery Training and Self-Help*, a relapse prevention manual for heroin addicts.

CONTENTS

FOREWORD

Group therapy is the most prevalent form of treatment for substance use disordered patients in both inpatient and outpatient settings. Group therapy has been used with alcoholics, opiate addicts, and more recently cocaine abusers because of its recognized ability to build cohesion among disenfranchised individuals and to address "core" issues of denial and rationalization that often lead to relapse among those with substance use disorders.

Despite its central role in virtually all substance abuse treatments and its potential for meaningful contribution to rehabilitation, group therapy with substance abusers has been poorly described and has been generally lacking in theoretical clarity or methodological sophistication. Further, group therapy has often been practiced in its most rudimentary form by poorly trained, irregularly supervised counselors providing helpful, but unstructured, and often aimless treatment in a group setting but without the essence of true group therapy.

With the development of Modified Dynamic Group Therapy (MDGT), through the Harvard Cocaine Recovery Project, Khantzian, Halliday, and McAuliffe have combined the important aspects of the traditional group setting with a rational and organized therapeutic approach derived from their decades of sophisticated thought, practice, and research with individual dynamic psychotherapies. These are among the only workers in the field today that could have accomplished this difficult combination. Their experience with substances abusers comes through clearly in the theoretical bases for the therapeutic approach. Their years of training and teaching of therapy skills is evident in the clear and well specified instructions supplied in this manual. There has been a need for a therapeutic rationale and a methodological framework that could bring better trained and more sophisticated practitioners into the field of substance abuse treatment. This manual provides both an organizing rationale and well described methods to meet this need.

ix

What is MDGT? As a therapy, MDGT begins from the position that substance use disorders start because of problems of low self-worth and/or the experience of negative affects and overwhelming feeling states. These qualities in turn provide "psychological vulnerability" to drug use plus the poor regulation of impulses and a lack of self-protection. From this view, the authors see the role of MDGT as providing insight regarding these qualities and a therapeutic situation and professional resources designed to instill and build normal defenses that would remove the underlying bases for continued abusive use of substances. As discussed in substantial detail in the manual, the role of the leader of MDGT is to direct his or her and the group's efforts at four therapeutic foci: (1) affect tolerance, (2) the building of self-esteem, (3) the discussion and improvement of interpersonal relationships, and (4) the development of appropriate self-care strategies among the substance abusers.

In terms of its basic procedural elements, MDGT is a rotating group membership treatment designed to last for six months in a series of twice weekly 90-minute group meetings. Group composition should be a minimum of three but optimally 8 to 10 members. MDGT is designed to be complementary to A.A. and to individual therapy. Absence from group sessions and lapses to drug use are considered issues appropriate for group discussions. Others rules of group membership are kept to a minimum, except for a prohibition against being high during group sessions. Prospective patients are interviewed in a pre-group session and in individual sessions; and those lacking motivation are self-screened out through early realistic discussions of therapy expectations. Seriously mentally ill or those in serious conflict or crisis situations are referred to other settings.

There are special requirements for the leader of MDGT groups. The leader must be a trained quite skilled professional who is able to be supportive, charismatic, and evocative in early sessions, instructive in middle sessions, and supportive and attentive in later sessions. Special attention is devoted to promoting insight by using the acute commonalities associated with problems caused by drug abuse, to lead to more substantive discussion about commonalities associated with the chronic issues of emotional discomfort and fears of vulnerability that may cause relapse to drug use. Clearly, this level of therapeutic sophistication is not for the novice.

The six months of group therapy can be roughly divided into three stages. In the early stages (weeks 1 to 8), there is a focus by the group on their lifelong attempts to harden against vulnerability. Here, the effort of the group leader is to have the group members learn to trust, share, and listen to each other. The leader does this by creating a tone of protection, not confrontation, and this is done by having the individuals draw on the commonalities of their acute experiences with drugs.

In the middle stages of MDGT (weeks 9 to 16), the focus is on attachment of the members to the group as a whole. The process is more active and reflective and self-protection gives way to self-expression. Special concerns during the middle stages of MDGT include turning acute issues resulting from drug oriented crises into realization that these issues are much deeper but less visible and that they have to do with chronic qualities of impatience and unrealistic expectations. Here, confrontation does come in but only when comments are made to devalue the group.

In the later stages of MDGT (weeks 17 to 26), the therapist helps to develop the senior group members into working therapists able to introduce the concepts to new members and to see not just drug use but other aspects of their lives in terms of their former personality structure. During the last part of MDGT, there is no longer an explicit focus on drug use, but on the self and the relation of personality structure to common problems that will confront every individual and which may provide reasons to relapse to drug abuse.

There are three major contributions offered by MDGT. First, this therapy integrates the techniques of *group counseling* in the treatment of those with substance use disorders (especially, but not exclusively, cocaine abusers) with *individual psychotherapy* for patients having long-standing problems of depression, anxiety, low self-worth, and impulse control. This acknowledges the complex and sophisticated problems of adjustment faced by substance abusers and brings to their treatment proven techniques adapted for use in the group treatment setting. Therefore, as a process MDGT is explicitly not designed to be simple nor is it suitable for application by novice therapists. It is designed to treat substance abuse by ultimately focusing on the long-standing problems of character and personality that are thought to lead to drug use.

A second and perhaps equally important contribution is that MDGT is suitable for use immediately after detoxification in patients who are in "early recovery." While it clearly emphasizes the need for safety and protection of the individual, these goals are seen as compatible with "insight" into character problems and their role in the initiation and relapse to drug use. The approach of this therapy is that the "central issues" of poor tolerance of negative affects and compulsiveness are important unifying aspects of personality that are capable of being addressed from the very outset and, if addressed sensitively and competently, are likely to foster long-term efforts at recovery.

Finally, MDGT offers an attractive alternative to traditional forms of group therapy for drug abusers. While it is designed to be compatible with these forms of therapy, MDGT offers therapeutic avenues that are simply not available in standard, peer-oriented counseling sessions. For example, in contrast to A.A., C.A., and N.A. where the idea is to "keep it simple" this form of therapy, as the authors point out, requires a deepening understanding of self and others and an awareness of complex group interactions and character structures in order to be effective. Further, unlike so many of the group therapies for substance abuse, MDGT is explicitly not confrontive. There is ongoing attention to building an atmosphere of safety and support and this may account for the ability of MDGT to retain up to 70% of its patients. Despite the focus on patient support and protection MDGT does not see these goals as being incompatible with insight into the problems of drug dependence. On the contrary, the view of MDGT is that fostering protection and comfort can lead to insight into the way character problems may lead to drug use. This development of insight is seen as a way to overcome denial and to strengthen abstinence motivation. This, in particular, is a major departure from interventions designed to address these issues solely through direct confrontation.

In summary, there has long been a need for sophisticated, professional involvement in substance abuse treatment. With the introduction of this manual incorporating both the rational use of guiding psychotherapeutic principles and excellent use of case examples to instruct the therapist, the field has finally gotten a structured way to provide this involvement. In this regard, this volume is not simply a theoretical discussion of the use of these techniques, but provides a good discussion of early dynamic theories, excellent treatment of substance abuse personality characteristics derived from 50+ years of combined experience of these senior authors, and provides both the explicit techniques and the rationale for their use. There is every reason to believe that this will be a standard in substance abuse treatment for years to come.

A. THOMAS MCLELLAN, PH.D., GEORGE E. WOODY, M.D.,
LESTER LUBORSKY, PH.D., AND CHARLES P. O'BRIEN, M.D., PH.D.

PREFACE

The aim of this manual is to define and describe the assumptions, focus, and method of Modified Dynamic Group Therapy (MDGT), a group psychotherapeutic approach which utilizes psychodynamic principles for the understanding and treatment of substance abusers. MDGT is designed to address addicts' difficulties in understanding and regulating feelings, self-esteem, relationships, and self-care which may predispose them to depend on cocaine and other substances. These four areas are the consistent focus of the treatment. The purpose of the manual is to provide guidelines and techniques for the important modifications of traditional psychodynamic group therapy which make possible the effective treatment of substance abusers.

We intend this manual to be used as a guide for experienced clinicians who lead groups for substance abusers. The therapist who can make optimal use of it is someone already well-versed in the addictions, psychodynamic theory and practice, and group psychotherapy. For experienced clinicians not yet familiar with the addictions, for students in clinical training, and for treatment staff knowledgeable in the addictions, but who do not have the requisite clinical background, ongoing supervision is necessary.

MDGT was developed as part of a larger study, The Harvard Cocaine Recovery Project, a National Institute on Drug Abuse-funded randomized clinical trial conducted at Harvard Medical School at The Cambridge Hospital since 1986. The Harvard study seeks to compare the effectiveness of two short-term (six-month) group approaches to each other and to a no-group control condition. Participants in all three treatment conditions receive individual counseling. The first experimental group condition is called Recovery Training and Self-Help (RTSH), and is based on a structured cognitive-behavioral, social-conditioning model of relapse prevention. The second experimental group condition is the model presented in this manual, Modified Dynamic Group Therapy (MDGT), a supportive-expressive psychodynamic group model adapted for cocaine addicts. The study seeks to compare the effects of the treatments on psychological functioning, drug use, and other significant outcome measures of the subjects at six- and twelve-month follow-ups. The Harvard study includes 214 cocaine-dependent persons from the greater Boston metropolitan area who volunteered for outpatient aftercare group treatment. Participants were solicited through television and newspaper advertisements and stories, radio announcements, agency referrals, and client word-of-mouth. A requirement of the research was to record the therapeutic approaches in a manual form so that the treatment would be consistent when therapists changed over time. This volume is our development of that effort.

The Harvard study signals a new interest in exploring the effectiveness of group therapy with substance abusers. At a national drug symposium in 1977, psychodynamically oriented leaders in the field concluded that group therapy presents too many problems, particularly that of treatment retention, to be used in a psychotherapy study. They indicated that individual therapy was preferable as the focus of such research (Woody, 1977). Woody, McLellan, and Luborsky (1986) also suggested that individual treatment is more viable than and better adapted to the lives of substance abusers than group approaches because addicts are less willing to self-disclose in groups and are resistant generally to group approaches. While these authors' work focused primarily on opiate addicts in methadone treatment, the persons in the present study were highly motivated cocaine addicts who volunteered for outpatient drug-free treatment. The Harvard study offers us a new opportunity to reexamine these important issues.

Length of time in treatment correlates highly with positive treatment outcomes. While many previous studies of substance abuse treatment were compromised by extraordinarily high dropout rates, the MDGT approach used in the Harvard study successfully retained nearly 70% of group members for the entire length of treatment.

Our experience in treating the severe addictions leads us to believe that group therapy is viable and offers many advantages over individual psychotherapy alone. A modified psychodynamic group approach that specifically addresses both the vulnerabilities and capacities of addicts enables them to stay in treatment longer and benefit more substantially than previously thought possible. We also believe that the modified psychodynamic approach described in this manual can be employed in the phase of early recovery from cocaine and other addictions once abstinence is achieved.

The approach described is a short-term group psychotherapy method tailored to the needs of substance abusers. While psychodynamic theorists often emphasize the severe preexisting psychopathology of all compulsive drug users and the difficulties of treating them, we emphasize the restorative capacities of these persons which allow them often to respond rapidly to a relatively brief group treatment. When given the opportunity to begin to understand themselves in the context of a safe, supportive, working group, we find that most group members, despite a broad range of psychological dysfunction, can maintain abstinence while in treatment and make significant psychological gains. This group treatment focuses on maintaining abstinence, coping with the psychological difficulties that underlie relapse to drug use, fostering a new understanding of oneself, tempering narcissism, and discovering that one can choose to think about and respond to life in less self-defeating ways. While a primary treatment goal of MDGT is to help the members recover from their addictions, it also seeks to initiate a process of psychological recovery from and repair of the vulnerabilities that precipitated and maintained the compulsive drug use.

This volume will define and describe MDGT, and discuss both how it is rooted in the psychodynamic tradition of supportive-expressive psychotherapy and the important modifications it sets forth to address the treatment of substance abusers. Also included is a clinical perspective on self-regulation factors in cocaine dependence, and a practical guide to the implementation of the MDGT approach, using detailed vignettes and transcripts of groups in different phases of recovery to illustrate techniques, technical issues, and the main themes that unfold during treatment.

Preexisting character pathology is not a criterion for exclusion from the MDGT group. We seek instead to welcome and prepare members for group, explain how the group addresses the urgent concerns that bring them to treatment, and offer a workable way to recovery. We exclude only people who are not abstinent, too disorganized to participate in group therapy (e.g., psychotic, acutely suicidal or violent, in severe crisis, or brain damaged) or those who continue to live in highly unstable situations (e.g., residing with a mate who continues to drink or drug). We emphasize the inclusion of as many addicts as possible.

Groups are powerful ways of addressing and modifying the vulnerabilities that lie at the heart of psychological suffering and compulsive drug use. Groups have the capacity, when well-led, to heighten self-esteem, to improve self-care, to oppose the forces of shame and isolation, to evoke the expression of individual character style, and to enlarge and enliven the person's view of self and capacity for choice. The MDGT group method makes available to drug addicts these same opportunities to benefit from psychodynamic treatment.

This is a clinical population thought by many to be not amenable to a primarily psychodynamic approach in early recovery from addiction, but who could only profit from such an approach much later in recovery. In addition, this is a group thought to be untreatable using psychodynamic approaches because of addicts' poor impulse control, fragile ego organization, and severe character pathology. Traditionally, they have been excluded from short- and long-term dynamic treatments for these reasons.

The mission of the Department of Psychiatry at The Cambridge Hospital since its inception has been to offer psychotherapeutic treatment to often underserved and excluded populations—the "untreatables," including the severely disturbed, the poor, minorities, drug addicts, and alcoholics. This Department supports innovative and nontraditional applications of traditional approaches to severe clinical problems. MDGT carries forward this spirit of innovation by offering a supportive-expressive psychodynamic group therapy for substance abusers.

ACKNOWLEDGMENTS

We are grateful to all of the clinical, research, and adminstrative staffs of the Harvard Cocaine Recovery Project. These include Sarah Golden, Vanessa Gamble, and Elizabeth Christie (three of the MDGT group leaders), Jeff Albert, Georgia Cordill-London, Tim Flynn, Lauren Goldsmith, Richard LaBrie, Elizabeth Stone Maland, Kum Kum Malik, Thomas McGarraghy, Elizabeth McMahon-Cicerano, Stephanie Pearlman, Michael Pelham, Hope Podell, Guillermo Rivera-Pagan, Susan Robel, Patricia Song, Linda Watson, Cynthia Webnar, Laura Wetterau, and Larissa Wilberschied.

The following Project Outreach staff were also of great assistance: Alan Chandler, Kevin McGrath, Rose Bernal, Paul Breer, Anthony DiPrimio, Glenda Kaufman Kantor, Todd Katz, Susan King, Richard LaBrie, Sherri Lewis, Kimberly McClain, Angel Mesonero, Susanna Nemes, Susan Nusser, Jim Ranahan, Beth Rosner, and JoAnn Scherer.

We owe special thanks to Sarah J. Golden, Ph.D. In addition to her major contribution to Chapter II, she read the entire manuscript at various stages, and offered many insightful comments that have been incorporated into the text.

A. Thomas McLellan, Ph.D., of the University of Pennsylvania and Philadelphia VA Medical Center, read an early draft of this book and made many important recommendations.

We wish to thank Seymour Weingarten, Editor-in-Chief at The Guilford Press, for his support and advice, and Rowena Howells, Managing Editor, for her editorial contribution which improved the book immeasurably.

This work was supported in part by grants from the National Institute on Drug Abuse (5 ROI DAO4418; 5 R18 DAO5271).

Groups, properly conceived and managed, are powerful vehicles for self-examination and growth. In reflecting on our personal and professional development and the important people to whom we are indebted, we are struck by how many of them had influenced us in the context of small group experiences. To a significant degree our enduring interest and belief in the efficacy of groups derive from the relationships we have enjoyed with many gifted leaders, teachers, mentors, colleagues, friends, and students in a variety of group settings. We believe they have helped us to find the best in them and ourselves in developing our ideas and contributions, especially in this book on group therapy. We believe that MDGT for substance abusers is an effective instrument for self-understanding, repair, and respect. For those who have touched and influenced our careers, we hope it will be evident where and from whom the special and beneficial aspects of MDGT derive.

For the first author (Dr. Edward J. Khantzian) these important relationships and group experiences span four decades. Emerson Schwenck, a Universalist-Unitarian minister, was the first to inspire and encourage me as a high school graduate in understanding myself and others and how charisma can be constructively employed. Around the same time, I was fortunate enough to meet and work with Kenneth Benne, benefiting from his enthuasiasm and understanding of groups, how they work, and how they bring out the leader in all of us. Subsequently, as a psychiatric resident, I learned from Elvin Semrad how the most central task for individual and group therapists is to help patients face and stay with their distress and suffering. Max Day was similarly important in helping to appreciate the importance of painful affect in the comings and goings of group experiences.

In 1966 John Mack founded and became the first Chairman of the Department of Psychiatry at The Cambridge Hospital. As his "point man" and co-founder of the Department I was able to enjoy and benefit from, since the beginning of my career, his special gifts in understanding and managing people in organizations. This was particularly apparent in the small founding group that formed early in our history. Subsequently, as a mentor, collaborator, and friend he has provided immeasurable support, guidance, and help in finding my way in the quest to understand and influence human troubles. His choice to build a Department of Psychiatry at The Cambridge Hospital was a good one. Over the years the Hospital and the Department, with their leaders and administrative staff, have been unique in their steadfast commitment to care for substance abusers. In this respect, thanks go to James Hartgering, Les MacLeod, Al Vellucci, and Melvin Chalfen. Also special mention of two people, Lee B. Macht, my dearly missed friend, and John O'Brien is in order. Their assistance as friends and their capacity to remain infinitely patient and supportive in their difficult roles as administrators are very important factors in this work. I am grateful, as well, to our current chairman, Myron Belfer, for his commitment to the highest standards of patient care and for maintaining and furthering the humanistic values and psychodynamic principles of the Department.

As with all organizations, there are many people who provide the administrative leadership and support without whom no group could survive. Highest on this list I place Helen Modica. Her constant presence, hard work on my behalf and that of the Department, and her advice and feedback in my organizational and investigative efforts have proven to be one of my mainstays. Donna Stone runs a close second as a special assistant, friend, and imaginative problem solver. Pat Carr, Donna Foley, Susan Mahoney, Michael Greene, Glover Taylor, Harry N. Hintlian, all in their own way lent important personal, material, and administrative support.

As we have indicated, The Cambridge Hospital and Cambridge-Somerville Mental Health Center have been singularly constant in supporting the drug–alcohol programs in Cambridge. One of the most notable aspects and spin-offs of these programs has been the special relationships they have forged with colleagues, collaborators and students. Jan Kauffman and Howard Shaffer come to mind, as do Al Corman, Rick Bickford, Robert Reid, Hilma Unterberger, Gerald McKenna, Bill Kates, Jim Beck, Bob Apsler, Mickey Burglass, Margaret Bean Bayog, John Renner, Kathy Babel, Bill Clark, Stephanie Jones, Nina Masters, Susan Miller-Havens, Carolyn Bell, Rob Schneider, Francisco Napolitano, and Joyce Levy. Collaborators who were and remain especially important are Lance Dodes, Catherine Treece, Hank Rosett, and Jancis Long. Norman Zinberg, much missed, and George Vaillant were also influential, less because we agreed with each other (which we rarely did), than, more importantly, because we respected and enjoyed each other. The staff on the "Special Team" at Metropolitan State Hospital deserve particular recognition for their devotion over the past two decades to dually-diagnosed patients, long before it was fashionable. Best and fondly remembered are Michael Levy, Sharlene Sargent, Jackie Michaels, James Fine, David Griffith, George Magrath, Florence Maddix,

Marilyn Feinberg, Ruth Saemann, Kathy Doller, and Jeff Speller; also so many of the aides and nursing staff over the years, too numerous to mention, but not forgotten.

Finally, I express my indebtedness, affection, and respect to a group of friends and colleagues who have influenced in important ways my interest in substance abuse and group work. My analyst, Sidney Levin, although deceased, remains in a special category. To Henry Krystal and Leon Wurmser I owe much thanks and gratitude. Their writings, friendship, and support have greatly sustained and influenced my work on substance abuse. Technical Review groups sponsored by NIDA and associations through APA, AAPAA, and GAP have allowed me to meet, befriend, and enjoy many esteemed and gifted colleagues who have also influenced this work. They include Bill Pollin, Jim Julius, Jack Blaine, Bill Frosch, Gene Kaplan, Rich Frances, Shel Miller, Bob Millman, Roger Meyer, Karl Vereby, Chuck O'Brien, George Woody, Tom McLellan, Lester Luborsky, Roger Weiss, Steve Mirin, Herb Kleber, Bruce Rounsaville, and Frank Gawin. And last, but not least, friends at the local level whose generous sharing over the years of their wisdom about and experience with groups include Jim Kirk, Bob Ferrell, Scott Rutan, Henry Grunebaum, and Norm Neiberg.

Kurt Halliday is grateful to the following people who have helped him in unforgettable ways: in New York, James Little, Frank Mulligan, Anthony Burry, Sharon Hogarth, Sima Weitzman, Jean Houston, Bernard Weitzman, and Bruce Paskow; and in Boston and Cambridge, Charles Ducey, Sarah Golden, Howard Shaffer, Alvin Becker, George Goethals, Paul Breer, Michael Levy, Doris Menzer-Benaron, Dan Brown, and the late Norman Zinberg. He also wishes to thank these special people in his life: Mark Halliday, Anne Condit, Liadainn Pearlman, his parents, Robert and Gloria Halliday, and most of all his wife, Carol, who gave him the time, encouragement, and love to complete this book.

This manual is the outcome of a project whose success required the dedication and hard work of many people. Dr. McAuliffe gratefully acknowledges the contributions of the clinical, research, and administrative staffs of the Harvard Cocaine Recovery Project. They created something quite unique. Georgia Cordill-London, the clinical director, deserves special thanks. The project's group leaders, individual counselors, research assistants, interviewers, secretaries, and administrators made this clinical research possible by doing their jobs so well.

The Department of Psychiatry of The Cambridge Hospital and the North Charles Foundation provided support for the study. Myron Belfer, Glover Taylor, and Helen Modica were particularly important in this regard. And the many treatment agencies, individual clinicians, and EAPS that referred their clients to us contributed in an important way to the success of the project.

Finally, the development of this treatment program was made possible only because there were recovering people who took a chance by participating in the project. Without their efforts to achieve recovery nothing that we did could have made a difference.

The service rendered by intoxicating media in the struggle for
happiness and keeping misery at a distance is so highly prized as
a benefit that individuals and people alike have given them an
established place in the economics of the libido. We owe to such
media not merely the immediate yield of pleasure, but also a
greatly desired degree of independence from the external world. For
one knows that, with the help of this 'drowner of cares' one can
at any time withdraw from the pressures of reality and find refuge
in a world of one's own, with better conditions of sensibility.

—FREUD (1930)

After a successful psychoanalytic treatment a patient is
definitely less neurotic (or psychotic) but perhaps not
necessarily more mature. On the other hand after a successful
treatment by group methods the patient is not necessarily less
neurotic but inevitably more mature.

—ENID BALINT (1972)

CHAPTER I

MDGT: An Overview

DEFINITION

This manual presents a model of group therapy for cocaine addicts based on the theory and technique of psychoanalytic psychotherapy. Both individual and group psychoanalytic psychotherapy assume that mental forces, such as drives and affects, operate within individuals beyond their awareness and that psychological structures and functions regulate these forces. It is the treatment relationship that activates and makes manifest the person's characteristic ways of thinking, feeling, and interacting. Psychodynamic treatment provides the opportunity for the analysis and modification of the individual's experience of self and others.

The approach described in this manual is based on a contemporary psychodynamic understanding of vulnerabilities in ego and self structure in addicted individuals in general and in cocaine addicts in particular (Wieder and Kaplan, 1969; Khantzian,1987; Khantzian and Mack, 1983; Khantzian and Treece, 1977; Krystal and Raskin, 1970; Milkman and Frosch, 1973; Wurmser, 1974). Our approach rests on the assumption that wherever there are psychological vulnerabilities individuals develop characteristic traits or characterologic patterns which attempt to compensate for, even as they reveal or betray, these vulnerabilities.

Much of the work of MDGT involves an examination of these traits and patterns as they emerge in the life of the group.

Over the past fifty years group approaches have been employed for the entire range of psychiatric disorders, particularly for character disorders and drug and alcohol dependence. The types of group therapy have varied widely in theoretical orientation, techniques employed, and explicit goals. For example, self-help groups such as Alcoholics Anonymous (A.A.), Narcotics Anonymous (N.A.), and Cocaine Anonymous (C.A.) are practically oriented. They view drugs and attitudes about them as the main problems, focus primarily on goals of abstinence and sobriety, and offer peer support. Other group approaches are based on cognitive-behavioral psychology and social learning theory, and center on modification of the drug-taking and drug-related behaviors. Relapse prevention techniques, environmental change, and extinction of drug conditioning are emphasized in these treatment strategies. Again, it is the behaviors related to habitual drug use rather than the person using the drug which are the central emphasis of this approach. In this paradigm, drug use does not necessarily reflect preexisting psychopathology. In contrast to self-help and behavioral approaches, psychodynamic conceptualizations locate the etiology and maintenance of compulsive drug abuse in the vulnerabilities and characterological makeup of the person.

The most effective forms of psychotherapy, whether individual or group, combine elements and techniques which provide support and opportunities for self-examination and change. More traditional group psychoanalytic psychotherapy emphasizes analysis of the characteristic subjective reactions and defenses (transferences) which occur in the treatment relationship between the group leader and the other members. Clarifications and interpretations are made by the leader to produce insights into processes and patterns beyond the group members' awareness. In supportive group psychotherapy, greater emphasis is placed on fostering trust and connection among the members and leader, and a high priority is placed on maintaining an atmosphere of safety and comfort in which characteristic and self-defeating ways of seeing oneself are enacted and examined. One can begin to reflect on one's characteristic ways of thinking, feeling, and acting, and in place of the automatic response one can explore new views of self and responses to situations.

MDGT is a supportive-expressive group psychotherapeutic approach, which specifically addresses the needs and problems of drug-dependent individuals. These may be conceptualized as vulnerabilities and disturbances in four areas: (1) accessing, tolerating, and regulating of feelings, (2) problems with relationships, (3) self-care failures, and (4) self-esteem deficits. These are four central dimensions of how character structure manifests itself in everyday life for everyone—intrapsychically, interpersonally, and in the larger world. While these manifestations may appear to be transient or even contradictory (Donovan, 1986), the underlying characterological disturbance often remains stable. MDGT seeks to address this central problem of character regardless of its more ephemeral appearances. This therapy is designed to foster interactions which offer support, safety, and abstinence but also to provide opportunities for the group members to recognize, understand, and modify the vulnerabilities which otherwise continue to leave them susceptible to drug use.

Ultimately, we view the treatment of character disorder as the road to recovery from addiction. Such a treatment strategy, though, demands a continued attention to and concern about maintaining abstinence and avoiding a relapse to drugs and alcohol. Once abstinence is achieved, character structure is thrown into sharper relief (Knight, 1972), and becomes more available to examination, understanding, and repair. While it is the drug-taking that initially brings the person to treatment, it is the treatment of character that leads not only to giving up drugs but also to a profound change in one's experience of self and the world.

We differ from other theorists (Bean, 1984; Flores, 1988; Brown and Yalom, 1977) who argue that no psychotherapy is advisable or possible for addicts in early recovery due to neurological deficits, affective instability, and the primacy of the need to focus on relapse prevention. While acknowledging these genuine difficulties, we nevertheless believe that once abstinence is established we can offer a modified dynamic group treatment which can sustain the person even in early recovery, lessen the potential for relapse, and lead to meaningful characterologic insight and enhanced self-regulation during and beyond the group treatment. Moreover, there is a higher degree of variability with cocaine addicts in the cognitive disruption and affective instability than there is for addicts in general and alcoholics in particular. By emphasizing safety, comfort, and control the MDGT approach allows for these disruptive factors, and thus, from the outset can be therapeutic.

MDGT's conceptualization of dynamic psychotherapy differs in its basic assumptions from early theoretical psychodynamic approaches to the understanding and treatment of substance abusers. In contrast to conceptualizations of psychotherapy that stress instinctual strivings, conflicts, and pleasure-seeking, we emphasize the developmental and structural impairments that have affected the addict's capacities for self-regulation. We see the main problem in most compulsive drug use as the addict's self-medication of psychological suffering, in the context of an inability to tolerate and regulate affects, take care of oneself, or manage relationships effectively. Such individuals also suffer from an impaired self-concept.

In contrast to other dynamic theorists, such as Meissner (1986) and Wurmser (1978), who emphasize the severe preexisting pathology of the addict, we also recognize and emphasize the strengths and restorative capacities of the addict which make therapy and recovery possible. We regard the addict as wounded, but at the same time as one who has a psychological foundation that is sufficiently intact to build upon.

We offer a reconceptualization of psychodynamic group therapy which views the substance abuser as treatable using a short-term modified dynamic group approach, once the person has achieved abstinence. We believe that traditional psychodynamic approaches which emphasize uncovering techniques, early development, and analysis of transference are inappropriate for the person in the early and intermediate phases of recovery. But if one understands that dynamic treatment can instead be focused on creating an atmosphere of safety and support where individuals can begin to learn about themselves and the way their character structure works, then dynamic approaches are possible with addicts in early recovery. We emphasize the importance of structure, continuity, activity, and empathy in engaging and retaining substance abusers in treatment (Khantzian, 1981).

Rather than encouraging the expression of painful affects and the exploration of unconscious material, we see the core of MDGT to be an approach in which an active and friendly therapist, with the help of a supportive, cohesive group, encourages and facilitates members to look at the four primary dimensions of MDGT as they play themselves out in their lives and in the group. Through this experience, the group member discovers alternative ways of seeing, experiencing, and exonerating her/himself, thus allowing for greater flexibility and awareness of choice in her/his life.

By using group experiences and vignettes to describe the phases and techniques of MDGT, this manual will demonstrate how themes central to addicts' vulnerabilities repeatedly play themselves out in therapeutic groups. The group members are thus provided with ongoing opportunities to identify, understand, and modify the interactions that are central to their addictive vulnerabilities and characterologic patterns. The MDGT manual is modeled in part on Luborsky et al.'s (1977) manual for supportive–expressive individual therapy with methadone-maintained patients. They demonstrated that the psychopathology associated with addiction can be delineated and targeted, modified with treatment (i.e., substantial positive change), and that psychological improvement is also associated with a reduction in the use of prescribed and illicit drugs (Woody et al., 1986).

ASSUMPTIONS

This section and the one following on the focus of MDGT are intended to provide an orientation as to how the group leader and members function and interact to provide therapeutic benefit to the member. MDGT assumes that leaders are most effective if they adopt certain basic concepts about their role, the substance abuser in a group, the nature of addictive vulnerability, and psychological suffering.

The Group Leader and Members

The group leader in MDGT establishes an atmosphere of safety and support in which abstinence can be maintained. The leader facilitates member interactions which foster sharing, the comparing of experiences, and an expanding awareness of self and others. In MDGT for cocaine addicts, group leaders are trained to provide structure, to insure safety and comfort, and to key specifically on the members' character problems related to the fourfold focus on feelings, relationships, self-esteem, and self-care. While clarification and interpretation are provided, we equally emphasize empathy, involvement, and support.

A group creates a special interpersonal context of relationships and experiences among the members and leader which allows for examining and modifying members' problems. Groups can be powerful vehicles for reversing tendencies toward isolation and shame because they create conditions and opportunities to examine and correct them. Psychodynamic group therapy is designed to evoke salient representations of psychological vulnerability and their characteristic defensive styles (what A.A. calls "defects of character"). In group therapy the therapist is not the main or only curative agent. On the contrary, the leader constantly fosters the realization that members as well are aware, insightful, supportive, and understanding.

Notwithstanding an emphasis on an egalitarian mode, group leaders must also be aware of their special position in the group: the purpose of the leader is to lead (Homans, 1950). The leader will be the target of recurrent powerful needs which are central to addicts' disabilities and dysfunction. Given their special problems with self-regulation and substance abuse, addicts will often turn to the leader for comfort, protection, clarification, admiration, and guidance. Skillful group management coupled with the appropriate responses of the leader to these requirements, will balance the legitimate need for the assistance and support of the leader with the need for further exploration of these themes, and will lead to the discovery that members can also provide what is needed for themselves and each other. As is so often the case in psychotherapy, the timing of when to provide and when to explore is important, especially when the disabilities of addicts are considered. When the group temporarily becomes fragmented, overwhelmed, stuck, or inhibited, the leader will need to provide for its members what they cannot provide for themselves. The role of the leader is to create and maintain an atmosphere of safety and cohesiveness, and to provide active leadership through all the phases and inevitable crises of the group.

The Interpersonal Context

Although we have designed MDGT specifically to examine, modify and compensate for the deficits and dysfunction in the ego and self structure of addicts, our approach rests on group interactional principles that other authors have described for group therapy with alcoholics. These principles are important and basic to an appreciation of the interpersonal dimension of all group work. They are reviewed here as part of the foundation for a psychodynamic understanding of substance abusers in groups. In particular, works by Sands, Hanson, and Sheldon (1967), Brown and Yalom (1977) and most recently Vannicelli (1982, 1989) have been especially helpful in describing both the interpersonal aspects of groups and the techniques for intervention which promote understanding and change. Yalom (1974) and Brown and Yalom (1977) base their assumptions about group work with alcoholics on the following change factors: interpersonal learning, group cohesiveness, existential factors, universality, catharsis, development of socializing techniques, altruism, instillation of hope, imparting information, corrective family-like experiences, and initiative behavior. They add the following: "Group(s). . . help members overcome feelings of self-contempt, loneliness, alienation and disengagement, as well as help them understand and alter abrasive, maladaptive, self-defeating styles of self-presentation" (p. 428).

Brown and Yalom provide a list of "basic assumptions" for establishing optimal interpersonal conditions for the understanding of self and others. They argue that groups are powerful vehicles for human contact, personality change, and symptom reduction. The process is enhanced and accelerated by a discussion of here-and-now issues. MDGT builds on the interpersonal context to provide a more specific focus on addicts' self-regulation vulnerabilities and the associated characterologic patterns that predispose addicts to their general symptoms, and to the specific ones involving the drugs they choose or prefer.

Vannicelli (1982, 1989) takes as a point of departure the work of Yalom (1974, 1985) and Brown and Yalom (1977) to describe the special techniques she employs in group psychotherapy with alcoholics and adult children of alcoholics. She emphasizes a focus on the interpersonal pathology in group as a means for members to understand their maladaptive and self-defeating ways of relating to others.

Psychodynamic Group Psychotherapy Modifications

In order to help addicts understand their vulnerabilities, MDGT requires modification of both interpersonal and classical psychoanalytic techniques of group psychotherapy. These modifications influence each individual as well as the dynamics of the group. Unlike groups that focus primarily on interpersonal factors, MDGT places a greater emphasis on the understanding of one's structural or characterologic disturbances and deficits (Khantzian, 1978, 1980; Treece and Khantzian, 1986) as these disturbances emerge in the course of the group experiences.

In contrast to a more conventional psychoanalytic group where Wolf (1971), for example, argues that a psychoanalytic therapist should seek out the identification and expression of the person's uniqueness psychodynamically and developmentally, MDGT encourages identification of commonalities in the service of overcoming the feelings of isolation, aberration, and shame that are so common and detrimental in drug addicts. Although ultimately there are individual differences in each person's susceptibility to substances, there are enough common features central to individual members' addictions that the group's exploration of them helps both the individual and the group as a whole to devise protections and support against their susceptibility to relapse. Also, given that MDGT is designed for individuals whose problems may be life threatening, the group therapy requirement for safety becomes even more paramount. Accordingly, the modification of fostering a shared goal of control and/or abstinence as a requirement for treatment imposes a greater degree of homogeneity on the group members than is usually encountered in psychoanalytic group psychotherapy.

Finally, although our approach with MDGT aims to elucidate and modify individual psychodynamics, we employ a more generic conceptualization of "dynamic". This assumes that beyond individual psychodynamics, the structure, norms, context, and aims of any group will generate its own dynamics which cannot be explained or understood by the summing of the individual psychodynamics alone.

FOCUS

General

The pervasive drug problems in our society over the past twenty-five years have brought increasing numbers of persons to treatment. Psychodynamic assessment and standardized psychiatric diagnostic measurement have documented that substance abusers suffer identifiable distress and have problems in adjusting to external reality. The nature of their distress and behavioral problems have been delineated psychodynamically and shown diagnostically to complement one another. In our view the diagnostic findings represent indicators of their ongoing inability to regulate their inner life and external behavior. Our perspective is that effective treatment must be linked differentially to these disabilities and disturbances (Khantzian, 1985b, 1986). These disturbances in affect, self-regulation, and character structure which underlie addiction become the primary focuses of treatment once abstinence is achieved.

With Luborsky et al. (1977) we believe that treatment efficacy is improved when we narrow our focus to the themes that are central to substance abusers' reliance on drugs. These necessarily include relationships and activities associated with drug dependence. The focus of Luborsky and his colleagues is on supportive–expressive individual treatment and emphasizes two main issues: (1) the meaning of drug dependence, especially the factors which precipitate and maintain drug use, and (2) discerning the substance abuser's core relationship conflicts.

Luborsky et al. (1977) state, "the way the therapist gains understanding of the intra- and interpersonal context for the patient's symptoms is mainly by figuring out the core relationship theme." (pp. 14–15). They point out that this relationship theme is apparent in many different relationships and that the "core" theme appears in all of the patient's communications about the past and present, as well as in the treatment relationship (i.e. transference). In our experience it is even more apparent that the "core relationship" theme or pattern plays itself out in group treatment with other members as well as with the leader/therapist. Often this is more intensely expressed by some members than others. More often the group leader becomes the target of these relationship themes, which provides the group with a chance to see and understand how the theme plays itself out in the person's life, especially in the symptomatic patterns of drug use and related behaviors.

The focus on "core relationship" problems and patterns as described by Luborsky et al. (1977) and Luborsky and Crits-Christoph (1989) in supportive–expressive treatment is also a prominent focus of MDGT. However, we expand the group focus to include other key problems with affect life, self-esteem, and self-care. In our experience patients benefit from a focus on how the use of drugs interacts with subjective feeling states, relationship problems, and self-care disturbances.

The self-medication hypothesis (Khantzian, 1985a) suggests that the addict's drug-of-choice is governed by particular states of distressful affect and psychological suffering. In the case of cocaine addicts, they often struggle with the opposite problems of being anergic and/or over-energized. In addition to a significant incidence of depression, a number of studies have also documented a disproportionate incidence (i.e. compared to heroin addicts) of bi-polar and cyclothymic illness among cocaine addicts (Weiss and Mirin 1986, 1988: Weiss et al., 1988; Gawin and Kleber, 1984, 1986). They compensate characterologically for associated, underlying self-esteem problems by placing a premium on achievement, performance, action, and activity. We elaborate on these characteristics of cocaine addicts in Chapter 3.

We propose that the effects of cocaine help to overcome the states of anergia and depletion which are usually associated with depression (Khantzian and Khantzian, 1984), and may also augment a hyperactive, restless lifestyle and an exaggerated need for self sufficiency. Group leaders need to be alerted to the characterologic telltales of these vulnerabilities as they are played out in group, especially the characteristic attitudes and modes of hyperactivity, self-centeredness, and counter-dependence, which often alternate with expressions of passivity and isolation. In some instances the group leader needs to gently challenge, if not puncture, such defenses. At other times it will be necessary to exercise a containing, modulating influence, and perhaps even to help activate and mobilize the de-energized patient.

MDGT provides a context in which to identify and elaborate on these vulnerabilities, defenses, and maladaptive responses that perpetuate many of the lifelong problems of addiction, including those involving drugs. Group members are encouraged to observe and describe in themselves and each other how problems with recognizing and regulating feelings, relationships, and self-care, and the related characterologic defenses that they employ, are intimately related to their susceptibility to drug involvement and drug effects.

Affect Recognition, Tolerance and Regulation

The nature of affect disturbance that causes substance abusers to seek chemicals that alter their distress is complex. Group leaders and members need to appreciate them in order not to draw premature conclusions or grow impatient about the patient's feeling life and the related reliance on drug effects. A number of reports have underscored the defects and deficits in substance abusers' experience of their feelings (Wieder and Kaplan, 1969; Wurmser, 1974; Milkman and Frosch, 1973). The emphasis in these reports is on the defects in their psychological apparatus which cause substance abusers to experience emotions in the extreme, namely, feeling too much or too little. In this sense drugs are used as a "prosthetic", or as a remedy against a defect in affect defense/tolerance, distress, tension, rage, shame, and loneliness, and/or a readiness to respond with activity or passivity in relation to one's environment. In other respects there is much vagueness and confusion regarding their feelings, and so patients are unable to give words to them ("alexithymia") or hardly seem to have feelings at all ("dis-affected"). These patients defensively fight rather than feel (Krystal, 1982; McDougall, 1984). Furthermore, the drug-of-choice or self-selection phenomenon (Wieder and Kaplan, 1969; Khantzian, 1975) suggests that for many substance abusers certain kinds of feelings predominate which determine their selection. For example, some individuals with feelings of rage and anger find opiates to be appealing, other individuals with energy problems associated with depression respond to stimulants, and restricted, closed-off, counterdependent persons often find the softening effects of alcohol and sedatives soothing and appealing.

Appreciating some of these complexities can help substance abusers develop a repertoire of responses to these problems as they experience and process their feelings in group. In some meetings an emphasis on empathy, on staying with individual or group distress, might be of paramount importance and there might be a need to use such an occasion to acknowledge how such states lead to avoidances and/or drug craving and use. On another occasion group members and the leader might have to spend more time helping a person to understand the emotions that a certain life event might stir. Groups at these times help people to see that sometimes they even use the confusing and disruptive effects of drugs as a controllable substitute for their feeling life which they see as uncontrollable and even more confusing. At other times it is useful to point out to a patient how a specific affect state evoked in group leads to a craving for a very specific effect offered by a particular drug.

Self-Esteem, Need Satisfaction, and Relationships

Much of substance abusers' distress revolves around their inability to feel good about themselves and their relationships with others, themes that play themselves out powerfully in groups. In this forum the substance abusers often reveal how they have failed to internalize adequately that part of development which allows us to sustain the admiring and being admired experiences of childhood. Typically, early life experiences provide a sense that one can feel good or validated from within or that one can reach out to others easily, when necessary, for nurturance and validation. Deficits and disabilities in such capacities, which are so often present in substance abusers, produce extreme and uneven patterns in satisfying needs around dependency, self worth, and comfort. As a consequence, "they alternate between seductive and manipulative attitudes to extract satisfaction from the environment, and disdainful, aloof postures of independence and self-sufficiency that dismiss the need for others [and thus] leave addicts susceptible to adopting more extraordinary chemical dependencies to meet their needs and wants" (Khantzian, 1982, p. 28).

As we have already indicated, many of the interpersonal aspects of groups provide some of the "curative" responses in an ongoing way through such shared, universal aspects as ongoing support and acceptance and the installation of caring, respectful modes of listening and interacting. Beyond these general elements the group leader can be instrumental in fostering an examination of the self-esteem and need satisfaction issues that cause group members to characteristically assume such self-defeating postures as an attitude of self-sufficiency, a disavowal of need, bravado, and counterdependency (Khantzian, 1986).

Self-Care

Addicts are often accused or accuse themselves of harboring and living out suicidal motives given the dangerous and life threatening nature of drug-dependency. In our own work we have been more impressed with the self-defeating and destructive aspects of drug abuse as a reflection of a more pervasive impairment in the capacity for self-care and self-preservation. A developmental perspective enables us to identify how addicts have suffered with lifelong vulnerabilities around self-care. This is evident in histories pre- and postdating their substance abuse, and includes accidents and preventable medical, dental, legal, and financial difficulties in which there has been a persistent inability to worry about, anticipate, or consider the consequences of their actions or inactions. With regard to the drug use itself, it has been striking to see how little substance abusers worry about its meaning or fear its consequences. These lapses and failures in self-care are symptomatic reflections of deficits in ego psychological structures and functions that otherwise protect from harm and danger. That is, most people are fearful and apprehensive and therefore avoid the many aspects and elements of drug use that are dangerous, whereas addicts often fail to show such caution, or lapse all too readily into states of stress disorganization and regression (Khantzian, 1978, 1982; Khantzian & Mack, 1983).

Our approach is more interested in building alliances with addicts in order to help them learn about their vulnerabilities in self-care than in suggesting or pointing out that they are self-destructive or pathological. The group can cultivate an empathic understanding of a substance abuser's inability or periodic failure to exercise caution when he/she reports the typical mishaps, slips, and disasters that occur as a result of this problem. Just as often the patients can be taught to observe the characterological tell-tales associated with this vulnerability such as counterphobia, hyperactivity, aggressive posturing, denial of danger, and bravado. In sum, we place great emphasis on actively and empathically identifying the self-defeating and self-destructive consequences of their self-care deficits, and on how these deficits increase susceptibility to addictive involvement. We demonstrate that the group members have not necessarily intended to be destructive, but rather that their self-care susceptibilities have caused them lifelong difficulties in reacting appropriately to harmful and dangerous situations, particularly those involving drugs (Khantzian, 1979, 1985a, 1986).

SUMMARY

Clinical and empirical experience and knowledge accumulated over the past twenty-five years documents the nature of substance abusers' psychological vulnerabilities. These include disturbances in self-regulation, as well as diagnostic findings indicating the co-existence of depression, personality disorder, and alcoholism, and are part of what cause the symptomatic and behavioral problems of addicts. In our work we emphasize a fourfold focus on problems with affect tolerance and regulation, self-esteem, relationships, and self-care, and point out how drug-taking has served to self-medicate the psychological suffering that arose from these difficulties. MDGT provides a context for understanding these vulnerabilities and the related compensatory characterologic styles as they emerge during group interaction. The group leader and, progressively over time, group members examine the characteristic responses in each other that demonstrate the self-defeating personality characteristics and defensive styles which both betray and attempt to compensate for these vulnerabilities.

CHAPTER II

Modifications of Psychodynamic Group Therapy for Substance Abusers: A Conceptual Review

with SARAH J. GOLDEN

In this chapter we review the theoretical literature relevant to the development of modified psychodynamic group therapy with substance abusers. MDGT conceptualizes addiction primarily as a psychological problem in the psychodynamic, psychoanalytic tradition. Drawing on psychodynamic, brief psychotherapy, group psychotherapy, and relapse prevention traditions, MDGT is a psychological approach which offers supportive, insight-oriented psychotherapy to substance abusers. Since substance abusers traditionally have been seen as unable to benefit from expressive psychotherapy, our model offers special modifications of support, safety, and therapeutic style to make it more accessible to the recovering addict. Again in contrast to the traditions from which it derives, MDGT seeks to understand and effect change in charactero-

Sarah J. Golden, Ph.D., is Clinical Instructor in Psychology in the Department of Psychiatry, Harvard Medical School at The Cambridge Hospital. She is Chief Psychologist on the William James Unit at Metropolitan State Hospital, and was an MDGT group leader in the Harvard Cocaine Recovery Project.

logical patterns in a group setting. It is offered as soon as abstinence is established, during the stage of early recovery. This chapter will explore MDGT as a reconceptualization of psychodynamic theory and treatment for addiction.

MDGT: A PSYCHOLOGICAL MODEL OF ADDICTION

MDGT is based on a psychological model of addiction. It defines recovery in terms of psychological recovery (integrating a new, active view of self) and psychological relapse (falling back into old perceptions and passive views of self), de-emphasizing the drug and drug-related behaviors and focusing instead on the exploration, understanding, and recovery of the self. Past and current experiences are explored in the effort to shed light on present life situations and characteristic ways of managing life problems. Drug use is always considered in the context of the individual's difficulties with self-regulation, involving affects, self-esteem, relationships, and self-care; it is seen as a way to assuage and control psychological suffering. Thus, MDGT offers a model of psychological relapse prevention that derives from psychodynamic psychotherapy, builds on the supportive–expressive models described by Kernberg (1986), Luborsky (1984), and Wallerstein (1986), and then extends these models from work with individuals to groups.

MDGT may be seen as the intersection of different conceptual strands in current clinical theory: short-term psychodynamic therapy (both individual and group), supportive–expressive psychodynamic therapy, group therapy with substance abusers, and the concept of the "early recovery" period, a time usually considered to be nonproductive for psychotherapy or even harmful to the recovering person. MDGT requires us to rethink and re-articulate both traditional drug treatment approaches and the range of indications and contraindications for psychodynamic therapy.

We propose a model of therapy which focuses on the here-and-now, increases awareness of self and others in a group, enables the group members to envision alternative ways of being, acting, and choosing, and which engenders the self-repair necessary to overcome addiction and avoid a relapse to drug use. We also hold that a supportive–expressive therapy focusing on the four areas of self-care, interpersonal relations, management of feelings, and self-esteem is more effective with substance abusers than a purely expressive therapy which emphasizes deep exploration of the unconscious, evocation of intense affects, abreaction, and catharsis. Our model is consistent with Wolberg's description (1967): "Psychotherapy is no mining operation that depends for its yield exclusively on excavated psychic ore. It is human interaction that embraces a variety of dimensions..." (p. 137). We offer a contemporary psychodynamic group approach to relapse prevention which lies within the spectrum of supportive and expressive psychodynamic therapies.

As a psychodynamic approach MDGT proposes a psychological model of understanding addiction which is both developmental and adaptive. The addictive use of drugs is seen both as an expression of vulnerability or deficiency in self-regulation, and as the attempt to overcome this vulnerability. In contrast to earlier psychodynamic formulations which emphasized the role of repression, sexual and aggressive conflict, and the satisfaction of libidinal drives in the etiology of drug addiction, more recent psychodynamic theory emphasizes vulnerabilities in ego and self structures which regulate self-esteem, self-care, and the capacity to relate to others as the root of addiction.

In 1930, Freud described intoxication as a way to avoid "unpleasure" by escaping from the "external world":

> We owe to [intoxicating media] not merely the immediate yield of pleasure but also a greatly desired degree of independence from the external world. For one knows that, with the help of this 'drowner of cares' one can at any time withdraw from the pressures of reality and find refuge in a world of one's own with better conditions of sensibility. (p. 25)

Intoxication was seen as both a way to mediate the "struggle for happiness" and a way of "keeping misery at a distance" (p. 25). Freud's emphasis is perhaps less on pleasure-seeking than on the reduction of distress (to achieve happiness is a "struggle", and unhappiness must be kept at bay). In the same way, MDGT understands addiction as a way to manage and assuage psychological suffering rather than as a primarily pleasure-seeking activity.

Rado in 1933 emphasized the basic depressive character of the addict, the "tense depression" which gives rise to the impulse to use drugs: it is "not the toxic agent but the impulse to use it...that makes an addict of a given person" (Rado, 1933, p. 78). Fenichel, too, emphasized the "morbid wish to be drunkenly euphoric" rather than the drug-taking as the problem to be treated (1945, p. 385). Wieder and Kaplan (1969) focus on the person with characterological vulnerabilities who uses the drug as a "prosthetic" to temporarily achieve a better adaptation to life. Krystal and Raskin (1970) discuss developmental inadequacies due to childhood trauma, which result in the addict's inability to tolerate or even to recognize affects. In their view, drugs are used both to avoid certain feelings and to experience others. More recently, Khantzian's work (1974b, 1975, 1985a) describes the self-medication hypothesis which holds that addictions result when individuals seek to relieve the painful affects and suffering which derive from deficits in ego capacities, in the sense of self, and in object relations. For these writers the vulnerable and inadequate self is the central problem in addiction.

With Kohut, the focus of the vulnerability shifts specifically to narcissistic disturbances. Kohut (1977) describes this vulnerability as a "defect in the self" which can manifest itself in addiction:

> The narcissistically disturbed individual yearns for praise and approval or for a merger with an idealized supportive other because he cannot sufficiently supply himself with self-approval or with a sense of strength through his own inner resources...the addict...craves the drug because the drug seems to him to be capable of curing the central defect in his self....By ingesting the drug he symbolically compels the mirroring self-object to soothe him, to accept him...the ingestion of the drug provides him with the self-esteem which he does not possess. Through the incorporation of the drug he supplies for himself the feeling of being accepted and thus of being self-confident; or he creates the experience of being merged with a source of power that gives him the feeling of being strong and worthwhile. And all these effects of the drug tend to increase his certainty that he exists in this world. (pp. vii–viii)

The problem with the drug effect is that it provides only "fleeting relief" for the addict: the basic defect in self remains, and the escape to drugs is only an illusory cure.

Meissner (1986), summarizing Wurmser's conception of compulsive drug use, describes the affective concomitants of narcissistic regression: "The core problem in addictive states is an underlying depressive organization with the attendant dysphoric affects of anxiety and depression frequently accompanied by feelings of shame and doubt based on an inner narcissistic vulnerability" (p. 354). Wurmser (1978) states that the drug "answers to a wish to regress to that image and feel of the self which can do and be everything, gets everything and disregards boundaries and frustrations—yet merely in illusion....It is regression in the disservice of the ego, freed of the controls of the ego, an illusory form of control mastery" (pp. 24–25). With cocaine, for example, the narcissistically depressed person suffering from passivity and feelings of unworthiness can achieve a sense of active mastery, of invincibility and grandeur. Meissner (1986) describes the narcissistic crisis as leading to affective regression that is "overwhelming and total, accompanied by feelings of anger, rage, shame, guilt, boredom, loneliness, emptiness, or depression" (p. 343). The drug offers a resolution of the crisis by modifying the painful affects associated with narcissistic wounding and by "restoring narcissistic balance" (p. 347). The drug offers something the person denies or is unable to provide for himself, such as feelings of competence and strength. Here the real addiction is to a view of the self that is invested in remaining weak, incompetent, and helpless without drugs.

Theorists such as Meissner and Wurmser stress the severity of the psychopathology underlying drug dependence, which includes fragile self-organization, poor object relations and affect intolerance, and the vulnerability to narcissistic crisis and regression. While MDGT acknowledges these severe deficits, we emphasize as well the restorative capacities of drug dependent individuals not only to overcome their addictions, but also to heal their injuries, to integrate what has been fragmented, to bear their suffering, and to develop a more mature, interdependent adaptation to life.

While drug addiction has been called the "stepchild of psychoanalytic theory" (Crowley, 1939), it survives into the present as an important focus of psychodynamic theory. Contemporary explanations of addiction in the psychological tradition include post-traumatic stress disorder (Schiffer, 1988), re-enactment of a core relationship conflict (Luborsky, 1984; Luborsky & Crits-Christoph, 1989), and an interpersonal conceptualization (Rounsaville et al., 1985). While psychodynamic theorizing about addiction is alive and well, what has been lacking is the development of practical applications to translate theory into practice. In fact, substance abusers are often viewed as too disturbed, too unmotivated, or too crisis-prone to benefit from psychodynamic therapies. MDGT seeks to employ the traditions of ego and self psychology not only to explore the particular vulnerabilities which increase susceptibility to drug involvement, relapse and drug effects, but also to offer a specific method of treatment.

THE SUPPORTIVE–EXPRESSIVE TRADITION

As a therapeutic approach MDGT is part of the supportive–expressive psychodynamic tradition (Luborsky, 1984; Kernberg, 1986; Wallerstein, 1986). MDGT creates a climate and mode of interaction that fosters an understanding of self and others and, in particular, an understanding of the psychological vulnerabilities that can lead to drug dependence, and of the individual's capacities that can lead to recovery. To the addicted individual whose only option has been action or drugs we offer an alternative—the possibility of holding onto and understanding the distress. In the MDGT group the individual is recognized and affirmed, even after revealing secrets that have caused him or her shame. It is this power of the group to accept the person, even beyond the addiction, that provides the curative force. It is this acceptance that frees the individual from narcissistic isolation; only then is an understanding of self and others really possible. Fried and Fried (1980), describing group therapy with narcissistically injured persons, state that regardless of the "dose" of "pathological narcissism" in a particular person, there can be no improvement "without reparatory experiences of acceptance" (p. 50). They include as the "highest form of acceptance" the "refusal to go along with" narcissistic defenses such as grandiosity, arrogance, and indifference (p. 56).

In MDGT the climate of acceptance begins with supportive psychotherapy. Kernberg (1986) describes supportive psychotherapy as a process which aims to strengthen the patient's defenses by using suggestion, some clarification, and environmental intervention, but not interpretation. The basic technique is to explore the patient's defenses in the here-and-now, "fostering a better adaptation to reality by making him aware of the disorganizing effects of these defensive operations" (p. 155). Expressive psychotherapy, on the other hand, attempts to bring about the reorganization of personality through the uncovering, exploration, and ultimately the weakening of defenses. Interpretation by a neutral therapist is its mainstay. While Kernberg holds that expressive therapy can be effective even for more disturbed patients, he suggests that it must be "modified." Supportive techniques can be used in the initial stages of therapy, but since this compromises therapist neutrality, he holds it is then difficult for the therapist to move to a more expressive model.

The concept of a supportive–expressive continuum—one that moves from suggestion to manipulation to clarification and finally to interpretation—may best help us locate the "modified" psychodynamic approach that MDGT provides. MDGT clearly uses many supportive elements, including an "active exploration of the patient's life" (Kernberg, 1986), an emphasis on suggestion and clarification, and an active, not neutral, therapist. However, the ability to identify long-standing characterological patterns as they emerge in the group with other group members and the group leader, to understand their roots, and to demonstrate how drug use affects how one lives one's life all qualify as the types of insight which can be approached through further clarification and interpretation.

Wallerstein (1986), describing a wide spectrum of psychoanalytic psychotherapies for forty-two patients at the Menninger Foundation over thirty years, suggests that supportive psychotherapy, the process of strengthening defenses, is the most appropriate one for addicted individuals. However, he acknowledges that in clinical practice a "varying admixture of supportive and expressive techniques" developed as treatment was individualized for each patient (p. 686). "Blurring" of the supportive, ego-building, symptom-containing mode with the expressive, uncovering, interpretive mode inevitably occurred. It is the supportive element of therapy that is usually less well-defined than the expressive one. Wallerstein describes supportive therapy as that which provides a version of the corrective emotional experience with a therapist who is "a kindly, understanding, reality-oriented figure" (p. 693). The therapist provides reality-testing and re-education, which both supports and educates the patient "toward reality-oriented problem solving" (p. 694). Wallerstein concludes that Kernberg's attempt to clearly dichotomize "supportive" and "expressive" are "just not supported by the detailed case material" (p. 699). He states that the supportive part is necessary so that the expressive work can be "received and sustained" (p. 699). This is consistent with the MDGT approach.

Luborsky (1984) defines the "main, distinctive characteristics" of supportive-expressive therapy as: (1) "guidance by the manifestations of transference"; (2) understanding thoughts and feelings as the "vehicle for changing what needs to be changed" (expressive technique); (3) supportive conditions for the treatment; and (4) nonreliance on advice-giving (pp. 9–11). The goal is an increased understanding of the core conflictual relationship patterns, of which the patient may be unaware, expressed in "relationship after relationship, like a theme and variations on a theme" (pp. 17–18). The idea is to re-experience and to begin to understand relationship patterns in the here-and-now. This is accomplished through a helping alliance with the therapist. In MDGT, however, there is a greater focus on the recognizing of one's own character patterns and conflictual relationships with other group members, not just with the therapist. Luborsky, unlike Kernberg, does not see the supportive and expressive modes as at odds: "the supportive relationship will allow the patient to tolerate the expressive techniques of the treatment that are often the vehicle for achieving the goals" (p. 71).

BRIEF PSYCHODYNAMIC PSYCHOTHERAPY

A focus on present life problems, a "corrective emotional experience" (a re-experiencing of old emotional situations in present and favorable conditions), a high degree of emotional involvement by both patient and therapist, and the appropriate selection of motivated patients are highlighted by Bauer and Kobos (1984) as features of brief psychodynamic psychotherapies. MDGT develops in part from this reconceptualization of psychodynamic therapy.

According to Gustafson (1984), it is necessary to "locate what is wrong, develop the intensity, and foster the missing capability" (p. 936). Brief therapy is often called "focal" in that it concentrates on a specific vulnerability or fault and challenges the character defenses around this vulnerability (Gustafson, 1986). Theorists of brief psychodynamic psychotherapy such as Sifneos (1979), Malan (1976), and Davanloo (1978) stress the "relentless" nature of their work, which moves "from difficult, relevant questions to relentless interference with defenses" (Gustafson, 1984, p. 938). For this reason, perhaps, Malan (1979) excludes certain individuals, such as drug addicts, from brief psychotherapy. Addicts, like other acting-out, severely character-disordered individuals with rigid or fragile defenses, are not considered to be safe or appropriate candidates for intensive, focused, brief psychotherapy.

MDGT, however, holds that substance abusers, despite their often severe pathology, can make use of short-term, intensive treatment with an active therapist who focuses on the individual's long-standing difficulties with self-care, relationships, self-esteem, and affect regulation as they play themselves out in the present. One of the modifications made by MDGT is exactly this type of active leadership, combined with group interaction. These groups also offer specific modifications of classical psychodynamic and interpersonal group therapy, as well as of brief psychodynamic therapy: first, the group provides the safety necessary to work in the brief, intensive model; and secondly, the group provides an opportunity to focus not only on individual characterological patterns, but also to bring out the commonalities, the "common ground" shared by group members. Thus, MDGT creates a context of safety, support, and empathy, and provides a focus for pursuing its brief psychotherapeutic goals.

GROUP THERAPY FOR SUBSTANCE ABUSE

MDGT draws on the general concepts of group therapy as well as the particular expeiences of group therapies specifically designed to address substance abuse problems. Its main distinction is that it provides a relapse prevention model that emphasizes the psychological vulnerabilities in the personality organization of individuals that leave them susceptible to emotional reactive patterns which make relapse more likely (Khantzian et al., 1989). It addresses issues other than the cognitive and behavioral factors associated with drug relapse by exploring the emotional life of the individual and seeking character change; at the same time, it does not rely purely on interpretations of unconscious material, nor does it focus solely on the group-as-a-whole, on the individual, or on the interpersonal interactions of the group.

While abstinence and relapse prevention are fundamental to an effective MDGT approach, characterological insight and change are its ultimate goals. It is within the secure containment of the group that the individual's characteristic patterns of managing, interacting, and experiencing are addressed as they emerge. Of paramount importance to the successful application of MDGT are the establishing and maintaining of safety within the group, an active, empathic, and direct style of leadership, the development of the group members themselves as sources of insight, interpretation, and support for each other, and a goal of understanding the individual within the group context as well as the group members' common psychological ground beyond their addiction to drugs.

The superiority of group therapy for producing character change has been the recent subject of several psychodynamic theorists. Guttmacher and Birk (1971) describe the group as a "catalyst," which elicits a "multiplicity of transference feelings" yet at the same time provides safety for the open expression of these feelings. Guttmacher (1973) holds that the cohesion of the group provides "reassurance" even as it functions to penetrate "the ego syntonic facade of character problems" (p. 513). Fried (1985) describes how group processes "push beyond insight," producing "innovative behavior" in group members. It is the responses of other group members that "motivate a search for new forms of self-expression and prompt new strivings" (p. 3). The "startles and surprises" that always occur in a group dissolve resistance; each group member unexpectedly "encounters" many countertransferences, a "plethora of stimuli, responses, and interactions" (p. 4). In addition, "there is the questioning that old and childish outlooks provoke in other members so that automatic behavior patterns assume more readily a problematic appearance" (p. 4). The group offers "emotional attention," but "the accustomed patterns don't work" (p. 8), challenging group members to envision a new way of being. Fried sees insight as a result of the encounter with the others in the group, not of interpretation per se. New forms of psychic self-expression are tried out in the group and then practiced over time.

Recently, Anne Alonso (1989) described group psychotherapy as the "definitive treatment for producing character change" (p. 1). Group processes such as amplification "can lift the individual out of his/her syntonic range of defensive response to expose some heretofore less obvious parts of the self," thus allowing the group member to move "from narcissistic self-engrossment to object relatedness." She stresses the need for reciprocal interaction to occur in order for character to surface, and holds that this kind of reciprocity cannot take place in individual analytic treatment as well as it can in a group. In the group, she notes (like Fried) that the "cost of character defenses is illuminated and presents a conflict which can render the same traits dystonic and thus available to interpretation and change" (p. 8).

While the development of methods for providing short-term individual psychodynamic therapy led to similar short-term group approaches, for both individual and groups the same exclusionary criteria have prevailed where substance abusers are concerned (Bernard and Klein, 1977; Klein, 1985). Addicts are seen as too disturbed for "focal" group therapy, even though this is a therapy in which patients share problems in living around specific themes and conflicts, in which the focus is on ego-functioning and the strengthening of defenses in the here-and-now, and in which the leader is active and supportive (Goldberg, Schuyler, Bransfield, and Savino, 1983).

Other short-term group therapy models, while excluding substance abusers as possible candidates, stress rigorous selection of group members, structured pre-group preparation, and the rapid development of group cohesion. Cohesion, an attraction to or a sense of belonging to the group, is seen as analogous to the therapeutic alliance in individual therapy and as a "central mediator" of outcome (Budman et. al., 1989). The therapist is the "manager" of this cohesion (Budman and Gurman, 1988). In brief dynamic group approaches the therapist is directive, "energetic," and makes "simple, direct interpretations" until cohesion is well-established, at which point the leader steps back and turns the group over to the members (Poey, 1985).

The advent of brief dynamic group therapy coincides with a shift from a more individual focus (the individual analyzed within the group), to a more interpersonal one (Kernberg, 1983). Budman and Gurman (1988) emphasize interpersonal factors, not symptoms, in finding a "working focus" for the group. Poey (1985) states that the "formulation should emphasize the way in which the conflict distorts present relationships and may be played out in the group" (p. 336). MDGT is distinguished from primarily interpersonal group approaches (Yalom, 1985; Brown and Yalom, 1977; Rounsaville, Gawin, and Kleber, 1985; Vannicelli, 1989) which locate the central problem in the realm of relationships and use the group as a "special social microcosm" (Vannicelli, 1988). MDGT emphasizes character as it is played out both individually and intrapsychically and in the interpersonal context.

Specific group approaches for substances abusers stress the interpersonal focus in ways that MDGT does share. Spitz (1987) describes a therapy group for cocaine abuse as serving as an "interpersonal anchor," within which the patient first finds "emotional equilibrium," and then is able to face "unresolved life issues" as they emerge (pp. 167–168). Cartwright (1987) also stresses the interpersonal and sees the group leader as a facilitator who encourages the group to determine its own focus, so that the "group members seek to understand each other from their own perspective" (p. 953). Cooper (1987), who describes group therapy for substance abusers based on the model of substance abuse as self-medication, cautions that we must be aware of the narcissistic vulnerability of these patients. Even as their defensive acting-out behavior needs interpretation, so their real developmental deficits, which manifest themselves in impulsive behavior, require attention and/or containment.

Borriello (1979), although not writing specifically about substance abusers, suggests that for any group psychotherapy with acting-out patients, we "focus on their uniqueness." That is, we must recognize that they are action-oriented individuals, who usually come into treatment in severe crisis, and who seek to avoid the conscious experience of feeling. Therefore, a here-and-now approach in which present events can be linked to other similar situations, both past and present, is crucial. Stone and Gustafson (1982), discussing the problems of treating narcissistic and borderline patients in group, emphasize the uniqueness of the individual patients, from the different ways in which each person joins the group, to such questions as the different and perhaps contradictory needs of the various group members; the problem becomes how to move between support and confrontation or, more succinctly, how to confront with empathy. Fenchel and Flapan (1985) advocate dealing directly with narcissistic resistances in group, with the stipulation that the leader should leave these confrontations to the other group members, if possible. Other resistances to be considered in the treatment of the narcissistic patient in a group include group resistances (for example, the straying of the conversation to trivia and social events) and even the therapist's own resistance (for example, seeking admiration, fear of losing group members, or boredom).

These specific recommendations for working with the substance abusing, acting-out, narcissistic, or borderline patient in a group all require a safe environment in which the psychotherapy can take place. We need to modify standard approaches if the more vulnerable, traumatized, and resistant group member is to benefit.

EARLY RECOVERY:
WHEN CAN PSYCHOTHERAPY BEGIN?

Kaufman and Reoux (1988) in a review article on psychotherapy with substance abusers (mainly alcoholics) distinguish three phases of psychotherapy: (1) achieving sobriety, (2) early recovery, and (3) advanced recovery. These authors present the popular view that in the early recovery phase the focus should be on the "disease," using mainly a cognitive-behavioral approach that does not threaten or too strenuously confront the denial of the patient. Only in the phase of advanced recovery (after 1 to 5 years of abstinence) can the therapy safely shift "from supportive to reconstructive" (p. 207).

Bean (1984) makes the strong statement that grief work and psychological growth are "luxuries" compared to the urgent, life-threatening conditions produced by substance abuse, which often take between six months and two years to address. Zweben (1987), drawing on the work of Brown (1985) and Washton and Gold (1987), cautions against exploratory, uncovering work early in recovery. She sees the work of therapy as "assisting" in "the tasks of recovery" which take place in "sequential stages" and in which such interventions as early attempts to "salve the client's battered self-esteem may interrupt the move towards despair that facilitates surrender" and thus abstinence (p. 256). She does acknowledge the relevance of dynamically oriented insight in the early stages, but emphasizes that it must be focused. Levy (1987) goes further, proposing that alcoholic patients can benefit from a modified psychotherapy. He suggests that not providing psychotherapy for such individuals and the bias against such therapy may reflect negative attitudes toward patients who are often in crisis or "intoxicated and demanding" (p. 786). He proposes a modified therapy which initially focuses on the drinking, rather than insight, thus avoiding the danger of a collusion with the patient's denial which might occur if the "reasons" for drinking, instead of the drinking itself, became the focus.

Levy, however, does not go far enough. Like Bean and Zweben, he essentially adopts an "either-or" stance regarding safety and insight. MDGT does not see these as incompatible, even at the beginning. In other words, within a safe environment, insight into character and the overcoming of addiction can take place from a very early point in recovery. In fact, understanding can fortify the awareness of the role of drugs, address denial, strengthen abstinence, and actually set the stage for a quick rebound should there be relapse.

SUMMARY

MDGT, then, drawing on psychodynamic theory, especially ego and self psychology to explain addiction, proposes a group approach that is supportive and expressive, emphasizes safety and empathy, but works actively and intensively to address characterological patterns as they express themselves in the group in the here-and-now. MDGT lies within the mainstream of group approaches for substance abusers in its requirement of abstinence, its emphasis on relapse prevention, and its careful preparation of group members for the group experience. In its inclusion of acting-out, often severely impaired individuals in a psychotherapeutic process that begins in early recovery, in its attempt to prevent psychological relapse as well as drug relapse, and in its promotion of psychological recovery as well as recovery from addiction to drugs, it offers a contemporary psychodynamic psychotherapy for substance abusers.

CHAPTER III

Cocaine: A Clinical and Psychodynamic Perspective

Unraveling the etiologic equation in the addictions has important implications for understanding how biology and psychology intersect in governing human behavior. Technologic advances over the past three decades have provided breakthroughs in understanding some of the important biological factors in the equation, the discovery of opiate receptor sites and endorphins being the most recent exciting example. During this same period extensive clinical work with drug-dependent individuals has also provided a basis to understand some of the psychological factors which contribute to addictive behavior. A contemporary psychodynamic perspective, complemented by psychiatric diagnostic studies employing standardized diagnostic approaches, has produced findings indicating that painful feeling states and psychological suffering are associated with the addiction and appear to be important etiologic determinants (Rounsaville et al., 1982a,b; Khantzian, 1985a; Khantzian and Treece, 1985; Deykin et al., 1987).

This chapter will focus and elaborate on psychodynamic and psychiatric factors observed to be important in the development of depend-

This chapter is based on a presentation prepared for a Technical Review Meeting on "The Epidemiology of Cocaine Use and Abuse" held on May 3–4, 1988, at the National Institute on Drug Abuse (NIDA), Rockville, Maryland. It will be published in a forthcoming NIDA monograph.

ence on drugs with particular emphasis on cocaine dependence. The approach is based on the assumption that the clinical context and the in-depth study of individual cases are valuable sources of data in seeking answers and explanations for what motivates human behavior in general, and troubling behaviors such as the addictions in particular. Ultimately the explanations that will serve best in solving the etiology of addiction will be those that integrate data derived from the biological, social, and psychological perspectives. It is the aim of this chapter to delineate more precisely the psychological dimension of cocaine dependence from a psychodynamic perspective with the hope that this approach can shed light on and contribute to an integrated bio-psycho-social formulation of cocaine addiction.

PSYCHODYNAMIC THEORIES—OLD AND NEW

Early psychodynamic theory placed emphasis on a topographic model of the mind (i.e., unconscious vs. conscious), drive (instinct) psychology, and the symbolic meaning of drugs, but did not make distinctions between the various classes of drugs. Consistent with this early theory, the emphasis in reports by Freud (1905), Abraham (1908) and Rado (1933) was placed on the satisfaction of libidinal (or pleasure) drives, or, in the case of Glover (1932), on aggressive drives. In these early formulations the use of drugs and associated practices took on important unconscious and subconscious meanings linked to early "fixations" in which an individual might be expressing or attempting to work out unresolved conflicts over sexuality and aggression. Although much of this theory is outdated, these early psychoanalytic formulations were heroic and revolutionary at the time in their attempts to go beyond superficial explanations and/or moralistic attitudes to explain the troubling nature of addictive behavior.

Where early psychodynamic theory stressed that misguided or repressed drives are at the root of addictions, contemporary theory places affect deficits and ego dysfunctions at the heart of addictive disorders. A division of the mind into the unconscious, subconscious and conscious with an emphasis on repressive mechanisms has been supplanted by a view of the mind which is concerned with feelings, functions, and processes involved in insuring self-regulation and adaptation to reality.

In addition to suffering as a consequence of deficits in recognizing and regulating affects (feeling life), contemporary psychodynamic studies suggest that addicts suffer as well because of vulnerabilities and dysfunction in ego and the self structures responsible for regulating and maintaining self-esteem, self-care, and interpersonal relations (Wieder and Kaplan, 1969; Krystal and Raskin, 1970; Milkman and Frosch, 1973; Wurmser, 1974; Khantzian, 1987b; Khantzian and Mack, 1983). These contemporary psychodynamic formulations of addiction have emphasized developmental factors and an adaptive understanding of addiction in which the use of drugs represents an expression of vulnerability and dysfunction in self-regulation. The use of drugs by these addicts is viewed as an attempt to self-correct these vulnerabilities.

CLINICAL DATA

The treatment relationship is a valuable source of information and data in identifying and understanding both the psychological vulnerabilities of addicts and how such vulnerabilities might motivate a reliance on drugs. In the case of cocaine addicts, for example, the clinical context offers opportunities to explore how the powerful energizing and activating properties of the drug interacts with feeling (or affect) states, personality traits, and character to make continued or regular use more likely.

A series of diagnostic studies over the past decade, complemented by clinical observations, has documented co-occurring psychopathology predominantly involving depression and personality disorder in cocaine abusers (Gawin and Kleber, 1984, 1986; Weiss and Mirin, 1984, 1986). It is significant that in these studies, in contrast to studies among opiate addicts, there was a disproportionately high incidence of bipolar type affective disorder, and in the case of the Weiss and Mirin studies, a high incidence of narcissistic and borderline personality disorder. More recently, Weiss et al. (1988) have documented a lower, but nevertheless substantial incidence of concurrent affective disorder and a higher incidence of antisocial personality disorder.

Our main source of data, however, has been direct observation of and experience with patients in the context of the patient–therapist relationship, either in the clinical interview or in individual and group psychotherapy. Such contexts provide unique opportunities to understand how state (reactions) and trait (characterologic) factors in an individual play a role in the susceptibility to a reliance on cocaine.

Empathic appreciation of patients' feeling states and the analysis and understanding of characteristic patterns of relating and behavior are part of the bedrock of psychoanalysis and psychoanalytic psychotherapy. These clinical traditions instruct us that a great deal can be learned about what motivates mental life and behavior. Following the nuances of reacting and interacting in treatment relationships allows clinicians to appreciate how personality and feeling states interact and play themselves out with the therapist (and with other members, in group therapy), and how they parallel characteristic reactions and patterns in one's life. Such data allow for inferences about a person's strengths and characteristic ways of coping, but also about the basis of the dysfunction and failure to cope that affects various aspects of the person's life. Further, it can provide unique and valuable data in understanding how a powerful feeling-altering drug such as cocaine may be adopted functionally and dysfunctionally in an individual's attempt to cope with internal feeling life and to adjust to external reality.

Luborsky (1984) has recently summarized the psychoanalytic traditions behind the technique and principles of psychoanalytic psychotherapy. More importantly, for our purposes here, Luborsky, with Woody and associates (Woody et al., 1986), has successfully applied these principles to narcotic addicts, demonstrating that they benefit from psychotherapy, depending upon the degree and type of psychopathology present. In their manual for substance abusers, Luborsky et al. (1977) describe how core relationship conflicts emerge in the treatment relationship and provide valuable clues toward the understanding of drug dependence, especially the factors which precipitate and maintain it. The relationship themes are apparent in many contexts. The "core" issue, or the core conflictual relationship theme (CCRT), appears everywhere in the patient's communication; about the past, about the present, and in the treatment relationship. We have found the Luborsky approach equally valid and applicable in individual psychotherapy with cocaine addicts for understanding how their feeling states and personality styles contribute to their dependency on cocaine. Along the lines developed by Luborsky, we describe how modified dynamic group therapy (MDGT) for cocaine abusers can activate core themes in which group members can learn how certain feeling states, and relationship, self-esteem, and self-care problems precipitate and maintain cocaine dependency.

The following description of the psychodynamic factors which we have found to be important in cocaine dependency is based on clinical observations in individual evaluation sessions and treatment relationships, and in the course of group psychotherapy with substance abusers.

THE SELF-MEDICATION HYPOTHESIS

As a consequence of the widespread drug use and abuse in our society over the past twenty years, an increasing number of clinical practitioners have treated large numbers of drug abusers in their private practice, in public and private clinics, and in conjunction and collaboration with self-help programs. Clinical work with such patients has revealed that they experiment with many classes of drugs and often use more than one drug simultaneously. However, despite the use of multiple drugs, most patients report that they prefer a particular class of drugs. Exploration of the psychological makeup of these patients, based on clinical evaluations and empirical studies, indicates that they suffer from specific painful feeling states and psychiatric disorders which play a role in determining the class of drug that they choose. Wieder and Kaplan (1969) referred to the "drug-of choice" phenomena and Milkman and Frosch (1973) to the "preferential use of drugs" to describe this pattern whereby addicts discover that a particular drug suits them best.

Khantzian (1975) originally characterized the differential preference for drugs as the "self-selection" process and subsequently, as the self-medication hypothesis (Khantzian, 1985a). Khantzian based his description and formulations on a careful evaluation of approximately 500 patients he saw in a public methadone maintenance program and in his private practice. He inquired in detail about all the drugs they had used, the subjective effects they experienced, and the drug they most preferred. In almost every instance the patients understood what he meant and were able to describe which drug they preferred when he inquired what drug did the most, or was "king drug" for them. A corollary to this finding was that in a significant percentage of these cases patients spontaneously added that drugs other than ones they preferred were often despised or avoided because of their adverse and unwelcome effects. These observations offer support for the theory that individuals choose drugs for their specific ability to modulate affect.

More recently, Khantzian (1985a) reviewed and summarized clinical and diagnostic findings which support a self-medication hypothesis of addictive disorders. Although some of the earlier psychoanalysts appreciated the pain-relieving properties of opiates, stimulants and sedatives, Gerard and Kornetsky (1954, 1955) were among the first to describe more systematically how inner city, New York opiate addicts used the opiates to overcome painful adolescent anxiety and associated ego and narcissistic pathology. Subsequently, work by Wieder and Kaplan (1969), Krystal and Raskin (1970), Milkman and Frosch (1973), Wurmser (1974), and Khantzian (1974a,b) produced observations and findings suggesting vulnerabilities and deficits in ego capacities, sense of self, and object relations which cause unbearable psychological suffering and intensely painful affects. Addiction prone individuals discover that the psychoactive properties of drugs-of-abuse counter and/or relieve these painful states.

Partly as an extension of these psychodynamic studies and partly as a result of the development of standardized diagnostic methods, reports by Weissman et al. (1976), McLellan et al. (1979), Rounsaville et al. (1982a, 1982b), Khantzian and Treece (1985), and Blatt et al. (1984) produced diagnostic findings documenting the co-occurrence of depression, personality disorder, and alcoholism which supported a self-medication hypothesis of addictive disorders.

Opiates

The pain relieving properties of opiates are well-known, and from this knowledge we infer that their appeal must be based on their ability to relieve emotional pain in general. In fact, work with narcotic addicts in methadone programs and in private practice suggests that opiates have appeal because of a much more specific action and effect. A series of reports have revealed that narcotic addicts have had lifelong difficulties with traumatic abuse and violence, at first being victims and subsequently, often becoming perpetrators. Whether victim or perpetrator, they struggle and suffer with acute and chronic states of associated aggressive and rageful feelings which are disruptive and threatening to self and others (Wurmser, 1974; Khantzian, 1974a, 1982; Vereby, 1982).

Narcotic addicts make the powerful discovery that both the distress they suffer, and the threat they pose with their intense aggression are significantly reduced or contained when they first use opiates. Thus addicts have repeatedly described the anti-rage, anti-aggression action of opiates as "calming—feeling mellow—safe—or, normal for the first time." Our experience suggests that the problems with aggression in such individuals are in part a function of an excess reservoir of this intense affect—partly constitutional and partly environmental in origin—interacting with psychological (ego) structures which are underdeveloped or deficient and thus fail to contain such affect. On this basis Khantzian has concluded that narcotic addicts find opiates appealing because their anti-aggression action mutes uncontrolled aggression and counters the threat of internal psychological disorganization and external counter-aggression from others—not uncommon reactions when such intense feelings and impulses are present (Khantzian 1975, 1985a).

Sedative-Hypnotics

Sedative-hypnotics, including alcohol, have an effect opposite to that of the muting and containing actions of opiates. The psychoanalyst Fenichel (1945) quotes an unknown source that, "the superego is that part of the mind that is soluble in alcohol" to describe the disinhibiting or releasing action of sedatives. Although this effect may explain the appeal of alcohol as a social lubricant in Western cultures, or why certain tense, neurotically inhibited individuals might prefer alcohol, its appeal for those who become and remain dependent on sedative-hypnotics seems to be more related to deep-seated defenses and fears about human closeness, dependency and intimacy. Krystal and Raskin (1970) have suggested that this class of drugs has appeal because the drugs dissolve exaggerated defenses of denial and splitting, and allow the brief and, therefore, safe experience of loving and aggressive feelings which are otherwise "walled off" and leave such people feeling cut off and empty.

Cocaine

Cocaine addicts take advantage of the stimulating and energizing properties of cocaine to counter states of depressive anergia and restlessness, and to augment or compensate for the personality factors that govern them. In the subsequent section of this chapter we will elaborate further on these factors in cocaine dependence. Here we will only briefly summarize previous psychodynamic and psychiatric factors that have been implicated in cocaine dependence.

Given the energizing and activating properties of cocaine, it should not be surprising that it appeals to both high-energy and low-energy type individuals. In the latter case cocaine has been considered appealing because it helps to overcome the fatigue and depletion states associated with depression (Khantzian, 1975) and to relieve feelings of boredom and emptiness (Wurmser, 1974). For the high-energy, restless personality types cocaine may be alluring because it leads to increased feelings of assertiveness, self-esteem, and frustration tolerance (Wieder and Kaplan, 1969), or augments a hyperactive, restless lifestyle with its exaggerated need for self-sufficiency.

Recently Khantzian considered, from a psychiatric/diagnostic perspective, the following factors that might predispose an individual to become and remain dependent on cocaine: (1) preexistent chronic depression; (2) cocaine abstinence depression; (3) hyperactive, restless syndrome or attention deficit disorder; and (4) cyclothymic or bipolar illness (Khantzian and Khantzian, 1984; Khantzian et al., 1984; Khantzian, 1985a). A number of recent reports have presented empirical findings to support the above speculations and clinical observations (Gawin and Kleber, 1984, 1986; Weiss and Mirin, 1986; Weiss et al., 1988; Kosten et al., 1987).

SECTORS OF PSYCHOLOGICAL VULNERABILITY AND THE APPEAL OF COCAINE

General

In earlier reports there was a tendency to associate or equate drug dependency with severe and significant psychopathology (Wieder and Kaplan, 1969; Wurmser, 1974; Khantzian, 1974a, 1980; Khantzian and Treece, 1977). We believe that this emphasis in Khantzian's early work on severe psychopathology as a determinant of drug use was a result of seeing a disproportionate number of heroin addicts in a methadone maintenance program. In more recent years, while working with increasing numbers of alcoholics and cocaine addicts seeking treatment, we find ourselves considering the possibility that degrees and sectors of psychological vulnerability are involved rather than global and severe psychiatric disturbance. Rather than identifying major psychopathology, our work with alcoholics and now cocaine addicts has impressed us that degrees of human psychological distress and suffering interacting with other factors are the important determinants in cocaine's subjective appeal for individuals. Notwithstanding this shift in emphasis from psychopathology to suffering, our clinical experience continues to suggest that the more extreme cases (i.e., associated with psychopathology where the suffering is invariably greater) continue to serve as valuable guides in understanding the psychological underpinnings of drug dependence.

Sectors of vulnerability in personality organization appear to play a part in predisposing some individuals to cocaine dependence. In our experience, however, there is no one personality type or "addictive personality" involved which generally predisposes a dependence on drugs or on cocaine in particular. Although not exactly personality factors, terms such as "sensation-seeking, stimulus-seeking, and risk-taking" which are described as risk factors in certain populations (Kandel, 1980; McAuliffe, 1984; McAuliffe et al., 1987) come closer to describing how a personality trait or predisposition could be influential in certain behaviors and activities which are forerunners of addictive involvement. We hope to show that "sensation-seeking, stimulus-seeking", and other traits might be particularly important for certain cocaine addicts.

In the remainder of this chapter we would like to highlight four sectors of psychological vulnerability, namely self-regulation vulnerabilities involving affects, self-esteem, self–other relationships, and self-care. We hope to show how such vulnerabilities may be important in the development of a dependence on cocaine.

Affects

"Feeling life"—or affects— appear to be distressing for addicts on at least two counts. They either feel their distress as persistent and unbearable or they do not experience any feeling at all (Khantzian, 1979, 1987). In the latter case, terms such as "alexithymia" (Sifneos et al., 1977; Krystal, 1982), "dis-affected" (McDougall, 1984), and "non-feeling responses"

(Sashin, 1986) have been coined or adopted to describe this inability to experience or identify feelings in addicts and special populations. These recent conceptualizations have helped to clarify that dysphoria predisposing to addiction may be unpleasant not only because of painful affects such as anxiety, rage, and depression, but also because feelings may be absent, elusive, or nameless, and thus confusing and beyond one's control.

In cocaine addicts depression or depressive affect has been most frequently identified as a chronic or consistent source of distress which impels individuals to depend on the stimulating and antidepressant action of cocaine (Khantzian and Khantzian, 1984; Khantzian, 1985a; Gawin and Kleber, 1986; Weiss and Mirin, 1986; Kosten et al., 1987). The ability of cocaine to overcome the fatigue and depletion states associated with acute depression, to activate chronically depressed individuals to overcome their anergia, and to help the user to complete tasks and to relate better to others is indeed a powerful short-term antidote to the self-esteem problems associated with these states (Khantzian, 1975, 1985; Khantzian and Khantzian, 1984). In these cases, self-medication motives seem to play a major part in the initiation and continuation of a dependence on cocaine. Many of these patients predictably and understandably respond to and benefit from the use of tri-cyclic antidepressant medication (Gawin and Kleber, 1984; Rosecan and Nunes, 1987).

Not all cocaine addicts suffer from clearly identifiable depression. In fact, in contrast to earlier estimates that as much as 50% of cocaine addicts suffered from depression (Gawin and Kleber, 1984; Weiss and Mirin, 1986), a recent study reported this number to be as low as 21% (Weiss et al., 1988). In this most recent report Weiss et al., (1988) attribute this drop in the rate of depression to changing epidemiology and a corresponding change in the characteristics of patients seeking treatment. In support of this change, they also cite an increase of 16% in the diagnosis of antisocial personality disorder in this which in the previous (1984) study sample was virtually nonexistent.

Although the changing epidemiology could be a sufficient explanation for these shifts in diagnosis, the elusiveness of and confusion about affect experience could also explain why it has been hard for clinicians to identify, specify, or elicit the presence of painful or depressive affect in many patients and in cohort samples. It awaits further study to conclude, then, whether vague feelings of dysphoria or atypical depression not picked up by diagnostic approaches might also contribute to the seeking out of the stimulating or activating properties of cocaine. It certainly is not unusual in clinical practice to discover many patients who complain of feeling bored and empty, or who seem devoid of affect, and it could be that it is such a state of being that causes "sensation-seeking" or "stimulus-seeking" and could explain some of the motives of "risk-takers." Certainly the qualities of sensation seeking and risk taking are preferred modes for antisocial characters. They are also notorious for being out of touch with or acting out their feeling life. Along the lines proposed by Klein (1975) for borderline personality disorder, perhaps it also holds true that individuals with antisocial personality disorder suffer with "states of dysregulation of affect and activation" and that many such individuals overcome their often hard to identify mood and inertia problems with the use of cocaine.

Self-Esteem and Relationships with Others

Cocaine is notorious for producing a sense of well being within oneself and in relationship to other people. As one addict puts it, "Coke fixes the ego." Its energizing action produces a sense of empowerment that can enhance a state of self-sufficiency and make contact and involvement with others exhilarating and exciting. Sexually, the user, in the short run, may also feel increased arousal and potency, and a sense of being glamorous and appealing. It should not be surprising then that basic aspects of self-esteem and relationships with others are often interwoven in important ways with the fabric of cocaine addiction.

Problems with narcissism are often at the root of the self-esteem problems involved with drug dependence. Kohut and followers (Kohut, 1971, 1977; Goldberg et al., 1978; Baker and Baker, 1987) in their development of self-psychology have proposed that narcissism evolves or unfolds along certain lines and takes mature (normal) and less mature (disturbed) forms, as is evident in certain personality characteristics. Healthy narcissism is basic to emotional health and consists of a subjective sense of well being, a confidence in one's self-worth and potential, a balanced valuation of one's importance in relation to other people, and groups, and a sense of how one fits in the world (Mack, 1981; Khantzian and Mack, 1989). In clinical work with cocaine addicts we have been impressed by the fact that vulnerabilities and deficits around these themes have been particularly important in explaining the allure of cocaine. Although a majority of these patients have been very successful and/or high achievers, and appeared to be psychologically intact, we have been struck by how fragile their basic sense of self-worth has been. This was most apparent in relation to their exaggerated preoccupations with physical or intellectual prowess, major concerns about performance and achievement, exaggerated needs for acceptance and approval, and vaulting ambitions.

Despite this exaggerated striving, however, cocaine addicts are surprisingly uneven and inconsistent in the ways they express their needs and relate to others. They may be alternately charming, seductive, and passively expectant, or they may act aloof, as if they do not need other people. Their supersensitivity may be evident in deferential attitudes and attempts to gain approval and acceptance, but they may rapidly shift and become ruthless and demanding in their dealings with others.

Individual psychotherapy and group psychotherapy provide opportunities to observe the characterologic (or characteristic defensive) telltales of these vulnerabilities in self-esteem and in self-other relations. Cocaine addicts have great difficulty in being honest with themselves and others about how driven, ambitious, and needy they are for recognition and acceptance. For many cocaine addicts high activity levels and an action orientation, augmented by counterdependent attitudes, disguise their dependency needs. For those who are more passive and depressed, postures of helplessness and self-effacement conceal from self and others that they are similarly governed, but are temporarily or more chronically defeated. For yet other addicts, disavowal of need and apparent self-sufficiency offer characterological protection from the realization that one is not all-powerful, perfect, and complete. Such patterns are often startlingly apparent in group therapy interactions with cocaine addicts, where their hyperactivity, self-centeredness, and counterdependence often alternates with reactions of passivity, discouragement, and isolation.

Cocaine effects interact powerfully with the acute and chronic feeling states engendered by the characteristic needs and personality styles of individuals susceptible to cocaine dependence. Their tendency to be hyperactive, restless, and driving can be augmented and sustained by cocaine's energizing properties, providing such people with a chemical boost or fuel for this preferred style. However, the extreme measures and standards of performance that such individuals maintain are difficult to constantly achieve. A not uncommon consequence is that such individuals periodically become depressed or more chronically suffer with or ward off subclinical or atypical depressive reactions and states. It is not surprising then that they find the activating, antidepressant action of cocaine desirable and adaptive on this basis as well. As the diagnostic literature indicates, and as is supported by the above clinical observations, it is not surprising that there is a disproportionately larger percentage of cocaine addicts (i.e., compared, for example, to studies of narcotic addicts) who suffer from bipolar, cyclothymic, borderline, and narcissistic disorders. All of these conditions share a common tendency for action, high activity, and rapidly alternating moods—conditions in which the augmenting and/or antidepressant action of cocaine might be desirable.

Finally, consistent with these observations, certain individuals who are driven, hyperactive, emotionally labile, and evidence attentional problems, experience a paradoxical calming response to cocaine much like hyperactive children with attention deficit disorder respond to methylphenidate. In 1983, Khantzian reported on such a case involving extreme cocaine dependence which markedly improved with methylphenidate treatment (Khantzian, 1983), and Gawin and Kleber (1984), Weiss and Mirin (1984), and Weiss et al. (1985) have also identified such a subtype. Although this condition has been identified in only 5% of cohorts of cocaine addicts, this interesting finding further supports a self-medication hypotheses of addictive disorders.

Self-Care

Because of the dangerous mishaps and often deadly consequences associated with drug abuse, addicts are often considered to harbor conscious and unconscious self-destructive motives. The highly publicized and untimely deaths of popular athletes and artists suggest that in each of these tragic cocaine episodes the potential lethal consequence was known by the victim, yet that person was not deterred from using it. Are these examples of pleasure instincts overriding survival instincts or, indeed, could this be the "death instinct" in action, or are they instincts at all?

There is little in our experience, or much in the contemporary psycho-dynamic literature (Khantzian and Treece, 1977), to suggest that these apparently self-destructive behaviors are governed primarily by pleasure instincts or self-destructive drives. As we indicated at the beginning of this chapter, such imputed motives in addicts derive from early and mostly outdated psychoanalytic theory. As we have also indicated, evidence suggests that drug effects are sought less to produce pleasure, and more to relieve suffering or to induce or enhance states of well being. Along similar lines, our clinical experience suggests that the self-damaging and lethal aspects of addictive behavior have less to do with self-destructive motives than with deficits and/or deficiencies in a capacity for self-care.

The capacity for self-care involves a set of ego functions which are acquired and internalized during childhood from the parents' nurturing and protective functions. Self-care functions serve particular aspects of survival including signal anxiety, reality testing, judgement, control, and the ability to make cause-consequence connections. When optimally developed, the capacity to take care of the self insures that we plan our actions and anticipate events to avoid harm or danger. In adult life, healthy self-care is apparent in appropriate levels of anticipatory affects such as embarrassment, shame, fear, and worry when facing potentially harmful or dangerous situations (Khantzian, 1980; Khantzian and Mack, 1983, 1989).

Although we first discovered and described the self-care vulner-abilities in narcotic addicts (Khantzian, 1974a), we continue to be con-vinced that in varying degrees this vulnerability cuts across all substance dependency problems including alcoholism and cocaine addiction. However, as we indicated previously, rather than being a capacity that is globally or pathologically impaired, self-care functions in cocaine addicts appear to be more or less established though are subject to lapses or regression. Overall their self-care functions are only marginally present, and so addicts do not adequately consider the potential danger or harm involved in using cocaine. Also, considering how needful, driven, and ambitious cocaine addicts can be, priorities about achieve-ment and performance could override self-care functions and self-preservation concerns that may be less than optimally developed or established. Furthermore, the defensiveness around the self-esteem and relationship difficulties seen in cocaine addicts causes compensatory posturing—counterdependent and counter-fearful reactions—which also interfere with appropriate worry and concerns about self-protection and self-care.

CONCLUSION

In this chapter we have reviewed the nature of some of the psychological vulnerabilities that appear to be important in the development of a dependence on cocaine. Clinical observations and psychiatric diagnostic findings associated with cocaine and other addictions suggest that self-regulation problems involving feeling life, self–other relationships, and self-care cause subjective states of distress and behavioral difficulties. The combination of distress and behavior problems leaves people who suffer with such vulnerabilities at greater risk for seeking out and succumbing to the powerful psychotropic effects of cocaine.

This chapter has not concerned itself with the issue of the degree or mechanism of interaction with other etiologic influences such as biological (i.e., genetic and neurobiologic) and sociocultural (i.e., setting, drug availability, environmental stressors) factors. Our own experience has led us to conclude that the psychological vulnerabilities delineated in this chapter have been important determinants in the development of cocaine dependence in patients seen in a clinical context. It remains unclear and awaits further study to conclude whether or not such findings in clinical populations of cocaine addicts are unique to them, or whether there may be implications for understanding cocaine use and abuse in nonclinical populations. For heuristic purposes we conclude that psychological factors, as well as social and biological factors, to some degree, play a role in all instances of cocaine abuse. The psychological factors that we have reviewed in this chapter exist on a continuum and exercise a greater degree of influence in some cases than others.

CHAPTER IV

Orientation to Group

GETTING SET

Groups are difficult to join. Normal self-consciousness, inhibitions about exposure, and ordinary embarrassment are some of the factors which interfere with joining and becoming involved with others in group situations. All of these factors are heightened when a person begins to admit that he or she has become dependent on a substance, and are further enhanced by the fact that many addicts describe a lifetime of feeling excluded from ordinary experiences of belonging. The quality of a psychotherapeutic group experience often hinges on how successful the leader and the group members are in establishing an environment that feels safe and comfortable enough for self-disclosure and participation in ways that allow individuals to understand themselves and others in the context of group interactions and experiences.

The leader plays a special role in the initial and early meetings by communicating and evoking values and ground rules that will enhance and maintain the commitment which is necessary for the work of the group. As we have indicated, the work of the group begins with their getting to know each other well enough so that they can focus on the personal and subjective problems regarding feelings, self-esteem, relationships, and self-care which have left them vulnerable to relying on substances to face these life issues.

As a consequence of their sensitivities about self-exposure and self-exploration, attention must be devoted early in the group's history to preparing and orienting group members and establishing norms that will ensure that the group holds together and achieves the aims of becoming drug free and gaining an understanding of the psychological vulnerabilities involved in substance dependence. In this chapter we will review what the necessary ingredients are for preparing and orienting group members, placing emphasis on a positive, direct approach which acquaints members with the nature of group work and group process. The model described here is a rotating short-term open group membership one whereby each member participates in the group for six months only, and new members are continually joining. This model can be used for longer-term groups as well.

PRE-GROUP PREPARATION

Pre-group preparation for new members joining an existing group is beneficial in that it reduces premature treatment dropouts and increases their motivation for psychotherapy. The MDGT method of orientation was initially dictated by research concerns about minimizing no-shows and early dropouts. As many of the potential group members were new to treatment, we sought to familiarize them with the workings of a psychotherapy group especially adapted to address their specific psychological vulnerabilities and characterological stances. We have found this method to be most effective in helping them join the group, and rapidly engage and participate in the work of the group. Unfamiliar feelings of acceptance, understanding, and belonging are welcomed by individuals who often feel left out and automatically anticipate exclusion. This method of orientation can also be employed in other clinical settings with nonaddicted individuals, because of its capacity to lessen the natural difficulty of joining and staying with a group of strangers.

Another pre-group procedure developed at the Harvard Cocaine Recovery Project is participation in an outpatient detox group. This group helps stabilize cocaine addicts through the first several weeks of recovery, teaches them the essentials of getting off and staying off drugs, introduces them to the group experience, and offers the support of other addicts who themselves are just getting clean (McAuliffe and Albert, 1990). After participation in this intake group the person joins the MDGT group.

Before the MDGT group meets as a whole, the group leader meets with the new members in a group format in order to provide a brief explanation of the group process, to anticipate the misconceptions and resistances they may have, and to engage them actively in the treatment process as a collaborative experience. The goal is to shape members' attitudes to the group, establish rapport, and give them a clear sense of the work ahead. While such pre-group preparation can be provided by an individual counselor, we have found that meeting with the group before seeing the individual counselor serves as a superior way of engaging group members because people act differently in a group. In our program, the individual counselor and the group leader are different people.

The therapist's task in the preparatory phase is to diminish fears, clarify misconceptions, provide support, and discuss the MDGT group process. The therapist can play a critical role at this point in establishing optimistic and realistic member expectations regarding the efficacy of the MDGT group. The member's initial expectations of and faith in the therapist are positively and significantly related to his remaining in treatment and to favorable outcomes (Yalom, 1985).

In the preparatory phase the therapist acquaints the new members with the established ground rules, which include strict confidentiality, attendance and promptness, and abstinence from drugs and alcohol. In addition, information concerning the meeting times, length and location of group meetings, place of meeting, and duration of treatment will be presented. Any questions regarding ground rules or procedures can be addressed at this time.

The therapist will discuss with each new member the general benefits of group therapy for substance abuse problems, and how short-term groups can effect significant changes in a person's life, through a reduction of symptoms, increased self-esteem, and improved self-care and relationships. It can be emphasized that while the members of the group have different life histories, all share the same serious problem with cocaine or other drug or alcohol dependence, and thus will be better able to understand and help each other on the way to recovery. They will have important contributions to make to others from their own experiences as addicts, which include the difficulties in living which both result from and contribute to the use of drugs to solve personal conflicts. At the same time, however, it is important for them to know that the discussion of drug use and drug-related difficulties will not be the central focus of this group. Rather, MDGT will consistently emphasize the person's character structure and not the addiction or drug-related behaviors.

The new member will be told that the group focuses on common concerns and personal issues, that his or her seeking help is in itself a powerful and positive step, and that he or she will be working with others who are seeking help for similar problems. The group provides each member with a safe environment in which to examine and understand core personal and interpersonal problems, to begin to look at his or her life in a new way, and to explore alternative ways to handle some old problems. Here one hopefully will be better able to manage anxiety, depression, and anger, as well as negative feelings and thoughts about oneself.

The therapist acknowledges to the members that groups are difficult to join, and that it is natural and to be expected that they will feel some apprehension about talking with a group of strangers about highly personal and difficult issues, but also assures them that this will pass. The therapist tells the members that there will be times when they will be disappointed in or feel frustrated by the group, by other members, the leader, or themselves but that this too is to be expected, and what is required then is to resolve to stick with it, not take flight, and to discuss these problems in the group as they arise.

The therapist explains the work of therapy. Cocaine and other chemical abuse is seen as arising in large part from the need to cope with life's problems. Therefore, the real issue in drug use is not the drug or the drug-related behaviors but the problems of the person who uses drugs. Improved self-regard comes from being better able to recognize, tolerate, and manage feelings, to handle the challenges of everyday life, and to regard oneself more realistically and favorably. It is further explained that one of the central goals of group therapy is to help the members help themselves to achieve the strength and insight they potentially possess to live more effective, fulfilled lives by drawing on capacities in themselves and others, rather than on chemicals, to manage psychological suffering.

The therapist also uses this preparatory opportunity to ask the members what their personal goals for therapy are, as well as what life issues are the prime source of difficulty which need addressing. This questioning occurs in general discussions and allows group members to spell out the personal and interpersonal problems related to self-esteem, relationship difficulties, regulation of feelings, and self-care that interfere with their lives.

The basic tasks of this brief preparatory phase are to make the new member feel safe, welcome, and valued; to reduce fears and misconceptions about the group and psychotherapy; to outline the rules and expectations regarding participation; to set an optimistic, hopeful tone regarding the likely benefits to the member; to state what the focus of the group will be; to establish the right tone for the group; and to encourage members to begin to reflect on some of their difficulties in living with which the group therapy experience may help them.

ORIENTATION AND SCREENING
OF PROSPECTIVE MEMBERS

The screening process is designed to address the general problem of the high dropout rate of addicts in treatment, as well as the suitability of the individual for the group, and the capacity of the person to function in a group setting. In MDGT prospective members attend a portion of one of the group sessions, generally on the second night of the week if the group meets twice-weekly. Prospective members not only observe but participate in this meeting for approximately the first thirty minutes of a ninety-minute group. The leader asks them to introduce themselves and to describe briefly some of the problems which bring them to seek help now. Current group members then introduce themselves and describe how they were not long ago struggling with similar problems and how the group helps them to remain abstinent and begin their recovery from drug use and psychological suffering. This time generally leads to the emergence of themes that will be the focus of that session which will continue after the prospective members leave. If prospective members focus on drug use, the leader will shift the discussion to personal issues, deemphasizing and discouraging war stories and drug concerns. The mood is one of warm and friendly seriousness.

Prospective members are given the opportunity to ask questions and voice their concerns. Once the leader feels satisfied that the prospective members have a good sense of the group they are thanked for coming and asked to speak with their individual counselor or the group leader in the following days to discuss their experience in the group. The prospective member goes through a 3-stage process: (1) a brief introductory meeting with the group leader prior to observing the MDGT group; (2) an introduction to the actual group experience; and (3) a meeting with the individual counselor to discuss the group experience.

This method of introducing prospective members to the group puts them quickly at ease, allows them to become connected to the group, and provides them with a sense of the group therapy experience. This approach enhances the likelihood that the new members will remain in treatment because they are encouraged to become involved even before joining and therefore do not feel as threatened when they enter the group. Even a brief experience with a good working group can quickly dissolve misconceptions about group psychotherapy. The sense of being accepted and welcomed is ego-enhancing, and the opportunity to hear from other recovering persons builds hope. Existing members have the opportunity to play an important role by teaching the newcomers group norms and expectations, modeling the real possibility of recovery from addiction, offering encouragement and support, recalling their early recovery difficulties and doubts, and encouraging the prospective members to persevere during this difficult period of early recovery. This experience enhances older members' sense of progress in the group as they inevitably compare themselves with fledgling members. The leader, using this method, will find it much easier to make rapid assessments of the new members regarding their suitability for group, as well as a preliminary working formulation of character styles, central issues, and levels of ego functioning.

Prior to the start of the MDGT group the prospective members arrive to meet briefly with the leader if he or she is unfamiliar with them. The leader welcomes them, begins to get a sense of their suitability for the group, and assesses the likelihood that they will remain in treatment. This orientation procedure where the prospective members meet with the leader and then with the current group members appreciably enhances the assimilation of the new members when they eventually join the group. It also increases the likelihood that the new members will remain in treatment, lessens their anxiety, and increases their motivation.

For the first fifteen minutes the therapist informally goes around the room speaking with each person, gathering basic information, and making a rapid assessment of mental status, diagnostic impression, and suitability for supportive-expressive group therapy. Specifically, the leader seeks to assess:

1. degree of loss sustained through drug use
2. history and severity of drug and alcohol use
3. reasons for entering treatment at this time
4. treatment history and treatment history outcomes
5. psychiatric history, including current levels of depression and anxiety
6. suicidal and/or violent ideation
7. level of any cognitive difficulties and neurological dysfunction
8. impulse control
9. diagnostic impression (Axis I and Axis II), and degree of antisocial features
10. current and prior job status and education
11. level of motivation for treatment
12. knowledge of and attitudes about twelve-step fellowships .
13. interpersonal functioning, including living arrangements
14. strengths that can contribute to the group and sustain recovery from drug and alcohol dependence

Hypotheses generated during this brief time are further confirmed or rejected as prospective members meet and interact with the regular group members. An experienced clinician can make a rapid and accurate assessment of the items listed above without having to interview prospective members extensively. The leader will have a clear sense from this brief meeting of the suitability of prospective members for group. It is our experience that prospective members who are unsuitable for group are likely to self-select out during this orientation phase, and it is usually unnecessary for the leader to reject them outright. If this is the case, however, the leader meets with the person to discuss why group treatment is not recommended at this time, and makes appropriate referrals. Most often, we do not "reject" prospective members. Instead, we refer them to more intensive treatment, postpone admission to treatment until issues such as childcare are settled and, in a few cases, suggest different types of treatment.

The leader explains to the prospective members the nature of the MDGT group and how it differs from relapse prevention and self-help groups with which they may be familiar. The leader also informs the prospective members that all discussion in group is strictly confidential. What they choose to say and what they will hear from others is held in strict confidence. Violation of this rule will lead to ejection from the group.

After this pre-group meeting with the leader the regular group members enter the room, the therapist greets them, and asks the prospective members to introduce themselves. The brief clinical assessment continues as the group begins to interact. Sometimes a newcomer brings up a problem and appeals to the current members for help. At other times a regular group member describes what the group has meant to him or her. It is the therapist's role here to insure that the discussion is lively, includes both new and old members, and avoids premature disclosure of traumatic material or an excessive focus on drug use. The leader informally, yet systematically, continues the assessment of the prospective members, particularly their interactive and character styles as they begin to emerge in the group, and asks questions that were not addressed in the pre-group preparation meeting. The following questions are helpful in assessing the suitability of the prospective member, and are nonthreatening ways to engage the prospective member in this first group meeting:

1. *Where and with whom does the person live?* If far away, how will he or she get to group? How involved or supportive are family and friends?

2. *Is the person in crisis?* If crisis generally brings one into treatment, what is the nature and severity of the crisis that brings the person to seek help now? Is the person at risk of harm to self or others? Are there any apparent neurological difficulties, such as memory loss, confusion, or difficulty concentrating? (If some memory loss is present, it is a relief to the person to hear that this is very common during early recovery, and that it will likely improve over time.)

3. *What is the work situation?* How long has the person been at the job, and how stable is the work?

4. *How long has the person been using drugs?* How does the person see the problem? What is the role of alcohol or other drugs in his or her life? What is the longest previous period of being drug- and alcohol-free? What were the circumstances surrounding earlier relapses?

5. *What is the person's previous history with drug treatment or psychotherapy?* How does the person imagine treatment can help? Are expectations realistic? Does the person see treatment as a passive, mechanical, or magical process? Is the prospective member workable, and will he or she interact sufficiently well in the group so as not to be a major disruptive presence? Is the person interested in others, or overly self-absorbed? Is the person in sufficient pain to keep him or her in treatment? Is the person acceptable to other group members? Does he or she know existing group members, and will that present a problem for the two of them?

The leader stresses to the prospective members that since the MDGT group requires a significant commitment of their time for the next six months, it is important to decide if they are ready for this prior to joining the group, if accepted. While they may feel enthusiastic today regarding their recovery, they will inevitably find it a burden to maintain regular attendance. It is important that when that time arrives they do not drop out before the end.

After being satisfied about a person's apparent suitability for group membership, the therapist encourages the prospective members to ask the regular group members about the group and recovery. As the group matures this portion of the time becomes richer, with the leader playing a less active role, and the members an increasingly active one. They recall how hard they found it to enter and remain in treatment; how they have endured and thereby felt better; and how the group has been supportive and helpful to them in their recovery. This interaction gives the members a chance to play an important role, not only by imparting information and acting as role models of recovery, but also by gaining a sense of how far they have come, and of the valuable role they can play in helping others as they seek to help themselves.

Often in an orientation session a new member will speak of loneliness, anger, or social insecurity, and the role drugs have played in solving such problems. The leader can use this opportunity to wonder if others have had similar experiences or motivations, and in this way draw some of the quieter members into the discussion.

The leader always seeks to head off the premature revelation of traumatic material in these pre-group and orientation sessions, as well as in the early phases of the group. Also, no prospective or current member is permitted to monopolize the time. When this starts to occur the leader keeps a tight rein and states that it is important to hear from each person in the short amount of time set aside for this introductory meeting. When prospective members seek to compare this group approach with twelve-step fellowship programs or other treatment approaches, the leader responds by indicating how this approach differs positively from the ones mentioned, and does not conflict fundamentally with other approaches to recovery. (We support and encourage participation in twelve-step fellowship meetings.) The crucial task is to let the prospective members see this group as primarily a safe, supportive place where they can be helped to end their addiction and make sense of their psychological suffering.

If the new and old group members begin a discussion that seems valuable for all to pursue, the leader may go over the regular time by 10–15 minutes. At the end of the allotted time, the leader thanks the prospective members for coming and participating, wishes them good luck, and looks forward to seeing them soon to discuss their experience of the meeting. If a prospective member is in a severe crisis, the orientation group may offer needed assistance and support to the person as a form of crisis intervention. In the rare event that a person is decompensating, unusually agitated or paranoid, or in a life-threatening situation, the leader will take responsibility for arranging further assistance and interventions as needed.

The leader wants the prospective members to leave with a positive view of the the MDGT group as something that can be helpful and important to them, and a greater belief in their ability to manage effectively during this difficult time of early recovery. It is our experience that this brief meeting and assessment can provide prospective members with a rich personal experience, and a good sense of what the MDGT group is like. We hope that this meeting also lessens their ambivalence regarding continuing in treatment, and thereby reduces the risk of premature dropout. We have been surprised to discover how this model of introducing new members is not only not disruptive to the ongoing group, but actually helps existing members by enhancing their self-esteem, consolidating their own gains, and reminding them in a helpful way of their particular vulnerabilities.

THE EARLY MEETINGS OF A NEW GROUP

Overview

This section focuses on the formation of a new group. In this rotating membership model, even after a few meetings there will be an existing group, with new members coming for the orientation and screening as we have described above. Once there are at least three members the group can begin.

The early sessions of a new MDGT group focus on : (1) the introduction of the group leader and group members; (2) a statement of purpose regarding the group from the leader; (3) an explanation of how psychotherapy addresses the substance abuse problem; (4) the ground rules governing active participation, attendance, confidentiality, and abstinence; (5) the focus of treatment; and (6) the setting of the tone of the group.

Opening Statement by Group Leader

The following is a statement of how a group leader introduces her/himself:

"I'd like to welcome you all to our group. My name is... Tonight we will begin with introductions, then discuss the purpose of our meetings, set the ground rules and expectations for the group, and then talk about some realistic goals we can hope to achieve in the six months we have to work together. Let's begin by going around and introducing ourselves, saying something about yourself and what brought you here. (Make sure that every member gets a chance to speak briefly about himself; in the event one member monopolizes the group time, or prematurely speaks of highly-charged conflict issues, gently move the group back to the task by acknowledging the problem, but assuring him that there will be time to understand that problem better, but for the present it is important to go slowly, and give everyone an opportunity to be heard from)."

Purpose of the Group

After the introductions are complete, the leader reflects back to the members some of the common themes and concerns the group has just raised, pointing out that a group can provide safety, support, and understanding for others who share the same predicament. Leaders can adopt their own metaphors for introducing these basic and important themes. The leader then expresses some of the shared concerns and motivations for getting help:

> "The use of cocaine, alcohol, and other drugs has led to many problems in your lives. Our job is to work together to begin to understand how things got out of control and what functions drugs serve in your life at this point.
> "We will offer support for your recovery and give you a sense of a drug-free self by working together in an active way, making this a safe place where, when you are ready, you can begin to explore some of these key concerns, and discuss some of the main difficulties you struggle with. We will meet twice a week for six months, and that is enough time to achieve some of your main goals, to make the start of a good recovery, and to greatly increase your understanding of who you are, how you relate to others, and to consider more options in living a realistic, drug-free life than perhaps you thought possible not long ago. At first we will spend time learning about each other, and how the group works."

Explanation of Psychotherapy

The leader offers a frame for understanding psychotherapy, and begins to reduce magical expectations and anxious concerns. The leader can offer the following statement:

> "There is nothing mysterious about therapy. You get out of it what you put into it, and you will be able to do this by slowly talking about who you are and some of your difficulties, and giving feedback and encouragement to each other. It's hard work at times, taking the risks

of opening up to others and making ourselves vulnerable, but this is exactly what can be most helpful. All people are wounded, more or less, despite how they appear on the surface, and yet often we feel alone in our suffering and what seems to be our unique situation.

"Therapy is not some magic thing done to you. We are colleagues in this work. You know yourself, your history, your struggles, and what makes you tick. My job is to help the whole group and you understand yourself more clearly, including your relationships with others, how you manage painful feelings, and how you take care of yourself. We are not here to moralize or judge each other, only to support and understand your suffering and capacities for recovery— not only from drugs, but from the old, stale, repetitious, and self-defeating ways of thinking, feeling, and behaving. Relapse does not only mean picking up but falling back into old self-destructive ways of seeing ourselves and behaving. If you stay with the group and give it your best, you will become aware of new possibilities and choices, and how your life might be.

"Often you may want to talk about drugs and drug use because that's what brought you here, but just as it was easier in the past to avoid certain problems by using drugs so too it is often easier to talk about drugs than to stop and take a look at ourselves apart from the drugs."

Acknowledging Group Members' Anxieties

It is especially important and useful for the group leader to acknowledge openly anxiety about beginning group. The following serves as an example:

"It's normal to be anxious and concerned when you begin some new thing like this, and there's usually a tendency to think either 'I can't do it. It's too scary' or 'I can do it alone, and don't need others, or 'This group is not for me, I'm not like the others and I might as well get out now.' I urge you to talk about these concerns and to stick with it. It will be well worth your while to join together for the purposes of support, understanding, and change. It does take courage, strength, and humor, and each of you by being here tonight shows clearly you are interested in things being better for you."

Ground Rules

Similarly it is the responsibility of the group leader to lay down ground rules which insure conditions for the safety of the group and its viability:

"We will meet on [specify days and times of meetings]. We'll begin and end on time. You are expected to attend all meetings, and not be late. In case of illness or an emergency, please call ahead to let me know. Any pattern of absences or lateness will be discussed in the group, so we can understand together what is going on. No one will be permitted to come to the group high.

"Another important rule for the group is complete confidentiality about what gets discussed here. Nothing is to leave this room, and this is essential for us to work together. This is so that each of you feels secure about speaking freely."

As beginning members usually lack a strong support system and are in crisis, the leader can offer them some guidelines about what to do in an emergency. First, members can get each others' phone numbers, and be encouraged to call if they need to. If the crisis is urgent, members can call their local psychiatric emergency room. If the problem is less urgent, they can call their individual therapist during office hours. In addition, members are encouraged to attend A.A., N.A., and C.A. meetings as often as they need to.

Formulating Goals

The leader helps focus and provide structure for the members by encouraging them to discuss what they hope to achieve in group. This can be stated as follows:

"I'd like now to turn to you, and hear your expectations and hopes about this group, and for each of you to speak briefly about your individual goals in recovery and what obstacles you anticipate."

While the members talk about their goals, the leader listens for shared themes, such as regaining control of one's life, rebuilding a sense of self, restoring and renewing damaged relationships, and returning to reality.

He/she then reflects this common ground back to the group. This is the beginning of a basic technique and thrust of the work throughout the life of the group, whereby the leader identifies that common ground where the concerns of the members intersect, where cohesiveness grows, and where insight occurs.

If the members focus initially only on their drug use and their wish for recovery from drugs, then the leader should encourage them to speak of more personal issues, such as self-esteem, work difficulties, interpersonal conflicts, and problems of self-care. The leader might ask, "What is it about yourself or your life situation that you would like to see change?"

The leader thus emphasizes again that the purpose of this group is to focus on the meaning of the drugs for the members in their lives, and not on the drugs alone. It helps also to establish a climate of safety, support, and trust by acknowledging, but gently sidestepping, highly-charged material that may emerge at this point, stating that they have experienced much suffering, and that it is the hope that our work here can help alleviate some of that pain through support and understanding. It is important that members see they need not discuss, until they are ready, issues that generate intense shame and anxiety. So, the rule in the early groups is—Always Go Slow!

Setting the Tone of the Group

While the task of the group is serious, and self-disclosure painful, the supportive aspect of this modified dynamic work actually makes the expressive dimension more potent if it is properly paced and carefully conducted. The leader plays a critical role in setting the friendly, yet serious tone of the group, and in helping to allow a free expression of the members' playful banter and humor.

The foundation on which the group will build hinges on the cohesiveness of the members. Since in this beginning phase cohesiveness is low, it is the first task of the leader to create a climate where this can grow. Just as individual therapy requires a sense of fit, rapport, and alliance, so does group work demand a common bond and sense of liking between the members and with the leader. Besides taking the members seriously, showing respect and empathy, it is also imperative that the leader be friendly, and not take him or herself too seriously. When the group becomes humorous and good-natured, it is important that the leader not always be in a hurry to get back to "work," for this itself is a large part of the work. Laughter and camaraderie help establish and maintain cohesiveness. The success of this modality is to a great degree the result of a group of people who look forward to being together. It is critical then for the therapist in the early group meetings to set a tone that allows this goodwill and group culture-building to flourish.

Conclusion of the Session

During the last fifteen minutes of the meeting the leader asks the group members how they felt about the meeting, responds to any concerns that arise, and summarizes some of the key themes of the session. The leader then offers the group encouragement and support, remarking that they've taken the first step on the difficult road to the recovery from drugs and the possibility of a renewed life. The therapist then concludes the session:

"We will continue getting to know each other better and learn more about the group, how it works, and what we can accomplish at our next few meetings. I'm glad you're all here, and I look forward to our working together."

CHAPTER V

The Early Group: Setting the Course

MDGT is an active, focused, directive form of group psychotherapy designed to focus on cocaine addicts' problems with regulating their feelings, self-esteem, relationships, and self-care, and how these vulnerabilities predispose them to depend upon and relapse to cocaine and other substances. Because of this focus, and the preeminent need for safety and abstinence, MDGT is more structured and directed than traditional psychodynamic group psychotherapy, but to the extent that MDGT also attempts to foster a psychotherapeutic experience which allows for a natural unfolding and examination of a person's characteristic ways of behaving and dealing with his or her emotions, MDGT is also open-ended and explorative.

The group leader is active and directive in establishing and maintaining the central focus, but the group process is sufficiently unstructured to allow group members time to acquaint themselves with each other and to play out their vulnerabilities and unique qualities. Because the group membership is everchanging, the leader constantly monitors the phases in the group's development, characteristics, and composition, and makes an assessment of what is needed by the current group. Therapeutic support and the identification, understanding, and resolution of characteristic vulnerabilities are provided through the members'

spontaneous interactions with each other, as well as the specific interpretations of the leader when he/she identifies focal or salient individual
or group dynamics. As we have indicated, groups, if carefully conducted, are ideally suited for identifying and working out "core relationship" problems (Luborsky et al., 1977), but they are also effective and
beneficial in bringing to light how an individual's problems with regulating his or her feelings, behavior, and/or relationship difficulties,
precipitate and maintain drug use.

Dynamic group psychotherapies differ from cognitive-behavioral
therapies in that the latter focus on changing behaviors related to the use
of drugs like cocaine, and the social and environmental cues which can
lead to relapse. This treatment consists mainly of problem-solving strategies to help prevent relapse and change the addict's lifestyle. The
cognitive-behavioral method is often structured and didactic, and main-
tains a primary focus on learning new behaviors, without addressing
the person's character problems. On the other hand, the dynamic approach emphasizes internal subjective states and the psychological processes and structures responsible for governing these states. In dynamic
groups in general, and in MDGT in particular, the group leader assumes
special responsibility, early in the group's experience, for demonstrating
this focus on character, and the related modes of speaking and listening,
for the other members of the group.

The role and attitude of the leader—and, by example and encouragement, the roles and attitudes of the members—are evocative and facilitating, and are employed to help identify, explore, and repair each
other's vulnerabilities and characteristic ways of dealing with emotions,
relationships, and view of self which predispose them to drug dependence. Where cognitive-behavioral approaches instruct and impart information, dynamic approaches evoke and attempt to understand deeper
layers of the self, especially the injured and vulnerable self, to draw the
wounded, hidden person into the light of the group, and to begin the
process of healing by interacting with the other group members and the
group leader.

MDGT places a premium on the establishment of rapport with group
members, a climate conducive to disclosures, avoidance of moralization,
condemnation of drug use and addict lifestyles, and an acknowledgment of the members as valued and valuable individuals. Change comes
about through understanding in a safe atmosphere in which straightfor-

ward give-and-take can occur. This new understanding spawns a sense of stability and dignity, and an ability to perceive that there are options in the way one lives one's life.

THE LEADER

In contrast to traditional psychoanalytic group psychotherapy, leaders in MDGT are more active, directive, and focused in their roles. This is especially so early in the history of the group, but it also varies as a function of the degree to which individuals in the group or the group as a whole grasp and adopt the modes and focus of MDGT. Although examples and group vignettes in this and the following chapters (as well as in the later chapter on technique), spell out specific responses, topics, and themes, we emphasize here the central importance of the leader in setting and maintaining the tone and flow of the group.

Attitude and Role

The group leader, besides being active, is also firm but caring in his/her approach. Up to a point the leader is also permissive, for example, in encouraging and joining in the group's playful joking. The group leader's attitude of friendly curiosity, interest, initiative, restraint, and even playfulness, contributes to creating an atmosphere where people feel free to speak, and able to begin to bear the pain they have sought to avoid through strategies of self-medication and self-deception.

Attention and Types of Intervention

The group leader exercises a varying degree of influence in each meeting on what or on whom the group decides to focus. The principle of "shifting attention" (Wolf, 1971) has been used to describe how no one person remains the focus of interest in group therapy, but the term might also be used to describe how the group leader encourages the development of particular themes or content. For example, MDGT is designed to focus on vulnerabilities in regulating feelings, self-esteem, relationships, and self care, but it is also designed for these themes to emerge spontaneously as patients talk about their experiences and reactions inside and outside the group. The leader helps the group to focus on these vulnerabilities by clarifying any one of these themes and appropriately labeling them when a member or members are struggling with a problem that relates to one of these areas. Beyond labelling, clarification sometimes provides "words-for-feelings" when patients cannot do it for themselves; at other times clarification is provided through instruction and explanation by the leader. Over time, the members catch on to the importance of clarifying and labelling important themes, and they begin to provide this service for each other. However, the group leader still plays an important role by providing and demonstrating support, confrontation, and interpretation.

GROUP VIGNETTE #1

Support, Clarification, and Finding a Focus in the Early Group

Addicts have a tendency to alternate between the extremes of blaming self or others for the distress and suffering entailed in their addictive illness. These patterns often play themselves out in group interactions, especially early in the group's history. The leader can be pivotal in providing and fostering clarification, support, and understanding within the group, which over time allows members to practice and adopt new ways to deal with their distress and their understanding of their addiction, themselves, and others.

The following example from an early group meeting demonstrates how the leader may offer clarifying and supportive observations which interrupt the members' tendency to blame and externalize, and give some impetus for more cohesiveness within the group. Although in this example it is only the third meeting, there is already some evidence of cohesiveness and group formation from the banter and playfulness prior to the meeting and at the start of group.

Joe began the meeting by half-seriously lamenting that he wanted to leave to attend the Red Sox baseball game, a special game he'd "never get a chance to see." Although the group laughed, in a way it was a test of the value of group for all of them. The mood became more serious when Fred, a 30-year-old man with a long history of IV cocaine use, said that the warm weather caused an urge for a cold beer which progressed to thoughts of "having some blow." He wondered why and admitted he felt scared. Paul, a 21-year-old man who had recently been stressed about his girlfriend's abortion and whose mother had died from alcoholism when he was 16 years old, commented how quiet the group was—"even though there's more people, there is less talk." Bill, a 27-year-old extrovert who has been straight for eleven months, said, "It's because of the weather."

Al, a bright 39-year-old former physician, commented on how the new people in group change the group dynamics and added, "It's not surprising since addicts don't like any changes at all." With some encouragement from the group leader, Al expanded on this for awhile. Fred asked the group if they believed you are born with addictive disease, and an animated exchange occurred with some arguing that addiction is an illness and others arguing that it has to do with "how you grow up."

Bud, a new group member who is a 35-year-old tradesman and a new group member, said that his wife put it on a moral basis and did not see it as a disease. The group seized this theme and concurred that they all face this kind of disparaging attitude when dealing with friends and family. Jim, a 35-year-old hypomanic man went one step further, adding, "People think addicts are scum." Bud evoked a side discussion about changes and loss when he complained that his wife will not face her own alcoholism nor seek treatment. The group responded supportively with a number of people pointing out that when they began to change and get better, people around them did not like it and acted as if they had lost someone—someone to get high with.

Although the group is acting supportively here toward Bud and rallying together around him as he describes his wife's bitterness and distrust, there is an undercurrent of "us in the group united against them out there who do not understand the problem." At this point the group leader is faced with an opportunity and a challenge. The challenge is to preserve the developing sense of unity and cohesiveness around the "us-them" quality of the discussion, but at the same time to help the group work on the low self-esteem problems associated with their drug dependence which they attempt to attribute to the moralistic and shaming attitudes of spouses, employers, and others outside of the group. That is, the members harbor these attitudes about themselves and worry and wonder. At the same time they avoid these concerns by projecting them onto others: "Is addiction a disease? Am I responsible? Am I scum?"

At this point the leader responded to the disease—morality issue by proposing an alternative to these either-or responses. He said, "I wonder if we can look at it another way. It isn't necessarily a disease or a moral problem, but maybe using drugs is a way of coping with psychological suffering which we experience in our relationships with other people and within ourselves."

Fred introduced a new theme. He wanted to know why his brother started shooting drugs just after he had stopped. The group discussed this as a common occurrence and an issue with which they all struggled.

Leo, a man in his late-40's, who was a hard-core, inner-city addict for more than 30 years, then spoke to the group: "I want to change the subject. I went to court today." He proceeded to tell the group that he was happy that he got a suspended sentence and probation for possession of works. More importantly for him, he wanted to emphasize his behavior. He said that in the past he had always used drugs before going to court and today he had not. He went on to say that he had come to treatment not particularly interested in getting straight, but to restore his veins so he could begin to shoot up again some day. In the past few weeks something happened to him here in the group and he now wanted to stay straight. With his voice breaking gently, he told the members that the support of the group helped him, that in a way the group was inside him today, and he thanked the group for what they had given him.

Fred then spoke of how he had gotten the urge to shoot up cocaine two weeks ago and how this really scared him. He thought aloud, "What am I getting out of being straight?" The group, however, was still with Leo emotionally. He expanded on his remarks and spoke of being proud of himself today and how he enjoyed facing reality. Al responded to Leo by saying how hard it often is to do things on one's own, and added that the group is a place where "you can get a battery charge" out of seeing others face things.

The group leader chose at this point to congratulate Leo for his good outcome in court, but reflected out loud with Leo and the group that what was even more important was that Leo could face and sustain his distress without resorting to drugs, that he could draw support from others, and furthermore, that he could face reality. The abilities that the group leader reinforced here are those of bearing painful feelings, depending and drawing on other people rather than turning to drugs, and improving his or her self-esteem by mastering a challenge.

Although this group is remarkable for sustaining such important themes so early in its history, it is still important for the group leader to be active in identifying, clarifying, and supporting what the group members provide for and achieve with each other. The group leader sets the stage to underscore and demonstrate for the group what will best serve the members as they continue to explore and understand their problems as addicts, and to change and mature as human beings. For example, as he admires Al's penetrating metaphor of the "battery charge", he supports and gives permission to other members to be wise and understanding with each other.

In what follows, the group leader decides to take advantage of the group unity and cohesiveness to reach out to a silent member, Dan, whom he knows from a pre-group meeting with his individual counselor has recently been in crisis and suicidally depressed. This intervention is based on the leader's sense of the group's positive sustaining capacity at this juncture, and the observation that as this group meeting had progressed, Dan, although quiet, appeared to be in harmony with the group, and not as depressed as his counselor had described.

The group leader asked Dan, a 29-year-old former broker in a prestigious real estate firm, if he would like to talk about what had been going on for him, leaving some latitude for the member to decide if he wanted to open up or not. Dan answered "yes" and began by explaining he had been caught embezzling money from his firm to buy drugs. His employer had subsequently gone after him with a vengeance, attempting to follow him to new jobs to inform new employers of his malfeasance. He also explained that he thought he was about to lose his house because of non-payments on his mortgage, but had just learned that this latter problem was temporarily resolved. He emphasized that he was still upset about his employer's actions. Other group members provided support by sharing similar experiences and becoming angry at his employers. Leo offered, "Don't let anyone rent space in your head," and Fred said, "I don't care what anyone says now because I know I am straight."

The group leader then offered, "Dan's story is everybody's story; there is a past that doesn't go away just because you stopped using drugs, and you have to deal with it." Leo supportively reached out to Dan saying he didn't know if things would work out favorably but that he was glad Dan was able to "hang in there—which was good." Bill interjected, "We're not responsible for our addiction but we are accountable for our recovery."

Heartened by the support he derived from his first, dramatic foray into the group, Dan next disclosed that for the first time in four months he drank on the previous weekend, in the context of feeling very depressed, hopeless, and suicidal. He said he had several martinis after a bike ride and then fell asleep. With encouragement from the group leader, the group subsequently began to key more specifically on how often all the members opted to medicate their painful feelings, especially feelings of depression, based on Dan's elaboration of his long-standing feelings of low self-esteem and depression. They also focused on how poorly they take care of themselves when they have isolated themselves with their distress. Someone in this context remarked, "addiction is spelled L-O-S-S! but you get your self-respect back." Jim expressed futility about looking into the past for reasons for drug use. Bill rejoined Jim saying, "If we don't study history we are doomed to repeat it."

The group leader remarked that Jim was right in one sense that "there was not a single event, for example, from one afternoon long ago when someone did something to explain why we do now what we do. The objective here is to look at patterns in our lives from early on up through the present where we can see that these patterns are still alive in our relationships, how we regard ourselves, how we do or do not take care of ourselves, and how we deal with difficult feelings and situations."

By this remark, the leader supports Jim but also encourages him and the other members of the group not to oversimplify the effects of the past. Rather, the group leader encourages a process of self-exploration about how our current patterns of relating and behaving derive from the past, and more importantly how these patterns are evident in current problems with relationships, self-respect, self-care, and feelings. These problems are what make them vulnerable to the need for drug effects.

Although this kind of statement might generally be used throughout a group's history to facilitate self-exploration and understanding, it is an intervention which is especially needed in the early stages of a group experience. Placing the emphasis on character patterns rather than past events, and linking these patterns to a focus on relationships, self-esteem, self-care, and feelings helps the members to establish a frame of reference and a guide. In contrast to twelve-step fellowships, such as Cocaine Anonymous, Narcotics Anonymous, and Alcoholics Anonymous, where the ethos is "to keep it simple," in dynamic group psychotherapy a deepening understanding of self and others is encouraged. The guidance of these organizing themes helps to illuminate and bring into awareness the dynamics and character structure of the members and to explain the complex group interactions of the group.

This group meeting ended with the leader thanking the new members for attending. The lingering positive feelings about the group and each other were evident outside the building as the members remained a while longer, talking in pairs. The leader ran into Dan and spontaneously inquired how he felt about speaking in group. Dan said it was "great" and he was glad he did and he felt much better. The leader replied that the group was for everyone, and he was glad that Dan had opened up.

The extremely supportive tone of this meeting facilitated two new members being meaningfully integrated into the group. Sensitive material and information normally difficult to share were disclosed, which contributed to the evolving cohesiveness of the group. People listened closely, spoke empathically, and there was a shift from monologue to dialogue. The group was also insightful, understanding, and effective in dealing with a patient's first "slip" (relapse), and they effectively linked people's pain and struggles to problems and difficulties with feelings, self-esteem, relationships, and self-care issues.

Modeling and Group Norms

As the above vignette demonstrates, the group leader plays an important role in modeling and encouraging certain group norms and behaviors which foster group cohesiveness and treatment effectiveness. The leader also acts to inhibit and discourage other responses and behaviors which reduce the group's cohesiveness and effectiveness. The group leader serves as a model by trying out new behaviors with the members, by maintaining a nonjudgmental, open, and honest attitude. He/she is energetic, optimistic, hopeful, and self-confident; he/she closely follows group patterns, helps members reframe issues, and makes simple, direct interpretations. At the same time the leader forthrightly and unapologetically deals with disruptive and inhibiting factors such as absences, divisive pairings, and scapegoating. The leader heads off and redirects verbal abuse or attacks, while discouraging multiple conversations and premature or excessive psychological probing.

GROUP VIGNETTE #2

The Opening-Up Process, Self-Consciousness, and Shame

The group leader in MDGT must be flexible as the group unfolds. He/she helps to move the group and keep them on track, despite any attempts by the members to defocus the discussions away from themselves.

A leader can often be extremely helpful by encouraging an embarrassed, ashamed member to give voice to painful issues never before shared or acknowledged with others. This can be accomplished by tactfully disclosing and elucidating on personal reaction of his own that touches on the patient's experience. In the following instance the group leader sensed that a patient was having great difficulty talking about his inhibitions concerning his ability to interact with and relate to women without the use of drugs. The leader was able to help the group, as well as this particular patient, when he realized that the group needed to break through and move beyond the veneer of macho banter that had persisted as part of the group's early history.

In this hour, Leo, the man in Vignette #1, awkwardly and nervously speculated out loud that he doubted anyone in the group had greater problems talking to women than he did. He indicated that he had never related to a woman before without drugs. After a brief period of even more awkward silence, the group leader said, "I don't know about all of you, but at least I have had problems talking with women

I wanted to get to know." The leader's hunch that with his comment he witnessed a sigh of relief from Leo and the other members was confirmed later in the hour as members began to share how drugs could provide a "persona" of confidence and ease, especially in encounters with the opposite sex. One man said he was twenty-seven years old but emotionally he felt only fourteen, adding, "I'm a mess at dances." He said he had to work on getting confidence now in such situations, but with drugs he "got it immediately," again emphasizing how he was also shaky in his self-confidence when approaching women without the aid of drugs. Another man said he had been clean for three years but was afraid to see people, lamenting, "I was clean but not serene."

Toward the end of this hour, after members had more humbly and honestly shared their problems of shyness, shame, and embarrassment related to engaging other people, Leo seemed freer to expand a bit further on what it was like for him.

He said, "I could always meet girls while on drugs—but it was all over once I stopped drugs. Drugs take us out of ourselves to that person that was always in us—confident, able to speak, be social, to work—to do what's necessary. But it took drugs and alcohol to get us to that confident self."

This helpful unfolding and sharing of these painful experiences of self-consciousness in their meeting was likely a direct by-product of an open and honest expression of vulnerability in the group leader. It is an example of how a group leader acts as a role model around sensitive and difficult life issues which members more often than not share in common. In his/her manner of speaking, choice of words, or singling out an individual whose problems mirror those of other members, he/she can grant permission for people to talk about what needs to be talked about. In another instance the group leader might admit to fear in a potentially dangerous situation, or to normal reactions to the painful realities of life, to help guide the group to talk about troublesome situations or reactions they might otherwise avoid or not admit to in themselves, or to each other. Group experiences provide repeated opportunities to focus on how ordinary life experiences are frequently avoided, and therefore not mastered, when the more extraordinary solutions which drugs offer are adopted. When the leader demonstrates that he/she also experiences and does not deny such reactions, it becomes safer for the patients to admit to, share, and enjoy, often for the first time, more ordinary human emotions and reactions.

THE GROUP MEMBERS

Getting to Know Each Other

In order for members to support each other and understand the characteristic difficulties which precipitate and maintain drug abuse, they need to get to know each other. Although the duration of MDGT is limited, to some extent members must be allowed to set the rate at which they reveal their difficulties and participate in the group.

Self-revelation and understanding occurs in a context of comfort, familiarity, and acceptance. Starting with the initial introductions, the process of getting to know each other works itself out over time as members talk about their past and present experiences and their reactions to each other in the group. Group members in MDGT are given a fair amount of latitude and in fact are encouraged to tell their stories and reveal themselves in their own ways—that is, to disclose their "actual selves." The group leader works with the members to develop a climate that will allow them to articulate and the group to remember what each members' goals are. As individuals tell their stories and convey or cover up their distress, the leader and other members need to foster empathic-supportive responses and interaction. This is accomplished mainly through a respectful listening and accepting attitude. Furthermore, the group members share with the group leader the responsibility for minimizing and picking up on verbal and non verbal reactions that inhibit or detract from open communication.

Although MDGT sets certain foci of vulnerability as important determinants of addictive behavior, different members experience these vulnerabilities in varying aspects of their lives. For some, work or their relationships with their spouse or parents predominate; for others, conflicts with friends or peers, or in a love relationship loom large; and for yet others legal entanglements, injury, or illness might be the absorbing issues. Whatever the case, members eventually reveal deficits, dysfunction, and conflicts about feelings, self-esteem, relationships, and self-care. Such difficulties characteristically and characterologically play themselves out, inside and outside group, around themes involving work, family, and friendships that precipitate and perpetuate reliance on drugs.

Character Style and Traits

As often as group members reveal the bases of their psychological vulnerabilities, they just as often, and for long periods of time, remain defensive about these vulnerabilities and resist any awareness of their problems. Dynamic groups are excellent contexts for individuals to identify with each other the character styles and traits which mask and yet are symptomatic of their vulnerabilities. For example, problems with recognizing and verbalizing feelings are often masked by excessive preoccupation with activity and the logistical details of what happened around emotionally evocative experiences, which has been referred to as "alexithymia," members with shaky or low self-esteem and conflicts over dependency often adopt attitudes of disavowal and counterdependency; and patients deny self-care problems through counterphobic attitudes and activities. Again, members are encouraged by leader modeling and support to respectfully and tactfully point out the subtle and less subtle traits in each other, and to gradually explore with each other what heightens, aggravates, and evokes these qualities inside and outside the group. In so doing they gradually identify and understand the vulnerabilities that govern their character traits and styles. In some instances members will play out the character problems with each other, and the group leader takes the initiative in pointing out these traits and their origins. On other occasions a perceptive member may be more effective in playing this role.

GROUP VIGNETTE #3

Understanding Characterologic Defenses

In the following example the group leader and the other members focus on the problem one of the members, Al, has with expressing feelings. In this meeting the group tries to help Al become more aware of how he covers over and denies the importance of his connections with other people. It is an hour in which some of the members cast about for a clear topic of discussion, and after a few preliminaries, the group leader chooses to pick things up by turning to Al, an aspiring landscape architect in his late twenties, who comes across as rather arrogant and supercilious, but nevertheless likeable. Suspecting that some of his disparaging remarks in the previous group about the usefulness of group therapy reflected a characteristic pattern of denying his dependency and need for help, the leader asks him if he might pursue what he had said further.

> Al affects a cool and lackadaisical manner and is not immediately forthcoming. The leader asks him why he comes to group? He says, "I don't expect too much; mental health is a lifetime process." The group leader observes that he has been quiet—especially for someone who has so much to say—and wonders out loud with Al that perhaps it is due to some earlier criticism from the group (i.e., referring to the group's reaction to his seeming indifference). Al denies this. With a bit more prodding he begins to speak of "looking for awareness" but then goes off on a critical tangent about Narcotics Anonymous (N.A.) as a form of "brainwashing."

It is important to observe here that Al, albeit somewhat extreme in his manner, is not an unusual example of how off-putting and disdainful addicts in general, and cocaine addicts in particular, can sometimes be. That is, a disproportionate number of cocaine addicts are active, self-sufficient individuals who take advantage of the stimulating and activating properties of cocaine to augment their preferred, hyperactive, counter-dependent style of relating (Khantzian, 1979, 1985b). Although the leader to some extent and the other members to a greater extent betray some impatience in their reactions to Al's disdain and intellectualizing, they creatively use these reactions to good advantage.

> The leader raises an old statement of Al's about controlled cocaine use. Al says, "I don't see any reason why not" (meaning eventually he might again resume controlled drug use). He then explains his need to be in group as a result of a "character deficiency" which needs to be resolved and not because of the drug itself. The leader cryptically

replies, with a hint of disbelief in his voice, "If you get rid of the character defects then you can go back and use coke in a controlled way." To which Al again says, "I don't see why not." For a period of time, the group challenges him about controlled use which Al characteristically fends off and disputes by disparaging the merits of using outside assistance such as A.A., N.A., C.A., and the group to learn why he needs the help of others to control his vulnerability. He continues to attack N.A. and A.A. as brainwashing and persists in his belief that he can someday control his use.

Nora, the only woman in the group, speaks up at some length for the first time. She poignantly conveys how much her dependency on A.A./N.A. and the people in them helped her. Al seems untouched by her story or her concern and instead cynically dismisses all the cliches of N.A. and A.A. He insists that a drug cannot control a person's life and his loss of control was the result of "emotional immaturity—and the ambiguity of the world." Several patients laugh, picking him up on his own cliche (i.e., "ambiguity of the world").

At this point the group leader should be concerned, and he is, that the patient is defensive and manifesting in an exaggerated way his most off-putting character traits of devaluation and disdain for other people's experiences, feelings, and needs. The effect is to make people impatient, if not angry, especially when Al's seeming refractoriness is weighed against the members' and leader's degree of concern and wish to help. The somewhat derisive laughter at Al and his characteristic pretentious statement about his problem with "the ambiguity of the world" indicates that members are frustrated and angry, and a breakdown of empathic concern for a group member results. This kind of interaction is central to effective group work because it forces people to deal with the most difficult (and often most immature) aspects of another person. These at times mirror their own difficulties with self awareness which will leave them feeling frustrated and powerless. At the same time, these feelings of frustration can provoke the other members and even the leader to respond with less mature, unhelpful reactions.

The challenge for the leader and other members is to gradually help each other discover that for different reasons we all adopt a variety of protective shields in our personality or character style. We each need help to see that the shield is there in each of us and that with it we protect a more lost and vulnerable self. Over time, through the group interactions, we can identify and accept our vulnerability, and ultimately, we can yield and change the exaggerated characterologic defenses (i.e, the shield) associated with our vulnerability.

The group leader picks up on Al's term of "character defect," suggesting to Al that he uses mechanical and passive images to describe himself, namely, that there is something wrong with him, that it can be simply corrected or removed, and that he can then just get on with his life. Al responds, "It's something like that—I'm just not mature. I can't accept ambiguity and I don't know how to deal with a lot of things. I was sheltered all my life and so many situations feel dangerous to me."

The group leader reflects out loud that Al sees himself as "defective"—lost in ambiguity, but that cocaine removes the ambiguity. Characteristically, Al draws on an abstract metaphor about always feeling his life is like a yellow traffic light which he constantly runs up against, never quite knowing when or if to stop or start, never seeing a green light. The group leader points out to Al that he speaks and then withdraws and appears indifferent to his own statements and the group's reactions. One group member interjects, picking up on the traffic light image, "This guy doesn't know when to stop."

The group leader chooses to focus on Al's defective self-image; he asks him to be more specific and personal and wonders out loud how Al feels about himself. He says, "I don't feel, I only use intellectual defenses." The patient is very convincing about not feeling. The group leader then asks how he feels in fact when he says something and the group rollicks with laughter at his posturing. Al denies it touches him. The leader asks how it was at home when his father was lost in his business and ignoring him. Al replies, "I became a juvenile delinquent just to get attention." The leader says, "You learned as a kid to shut down your feelings." Al says, "No, not to shut down but to do something else instead." The leader says, "With your wife—or for that matter with the group—is it a matter of indifference if she likes you, or if we respond to you?" To this Al says, "I have to learn how to love."

In the preceding interaction the group leader uses his awareness of his own impatience, evoked by Al's style, to guide Al and the group to appreciate that Al (and others) must need such defenses because there is an injured or vulnerable self in need of protection. Although we see glimmers of vulnerability (and thus the basis of Al's defensiveness) as the leader and members persist, the members must also back off after awhile, which the leader allows, trusting that the relinquishing of one's defensiveness is a gradual process. Three weeks later (see Group Vignette #5, page 97), we can see a positive change in Al's attitude as a consequence of the persistence and patience shown by the leader and group members.

Resistance and the Process of Joining the Group

As we have already suggested, it is difficult to join and remain in a group. Resistance, therefore, is to be expected and not prematurely or excessively challenged, and patients are allowed a certain latitude in setting their own pace in joining the group. The character traits and defenses just described are usually heightened at the outset of group and are one of the main ways members manifest their resistance. The task for the leader and the group members in this early phase is to support and/or accept these defenses without imposing restrictive goals or premature confrontations on these resistances. Despite resistances, the group leader can adopt an active, directive, and even managerial style to demonstrate to the group members that they can relatively quickly form a cohesive group, become interactive and supportive with each other, foster a climate of mutuality, and begin an interactive phase of work which does not depend solely on the leader.

Group members usually come to appreciate how much of their drug reliance has been a consequence of dealing with feelings, character, and relationship problems through activity and action. The group leader encourages patients to appreciate how their ways of coping and the crises they precipitate are linked to the past; they need to acknowledge their painful feelings from the past and in the present, and to support each other in finding alternative ways to cope with their painful feeling states and problems in living. The group members are guided by the leader and each other to focus on self, to be curious about their motivations, and to become aware of their reactions, in the present, to the other group members and to the therapist.

The leader should specifically articulate that, given a past tendency to substitute action and activity for feeling, at some level each member will not want to come to group. This is a reaction to be expected but not enacted, and they will have to help each other focus on such maladaptive reactions and behaviors. Boriello (1979) highlights the important ways addicts use action, crisis, denial, externalization, and intellectualization to deal with life's problems rather than being able to reflect, delay gratification, and bear painful feelings.

The group leader and, over time, the group members, can continue to reiterate group mores that can counter these trends, such as following the ground rules, being accepted and acknowledged by the group over time, and becoming more aware of how one chooses certain situations and responses, and discussing what responses are possible.

Self-Esteem Maintenance

It is especially important that the group members share with the leader responsibility for respecting members' defenses by not prematurely or on any one occasion excessively exposing a member's vulnerabilities and shortcomings. Although it soon becomes apparent that drugs and alcohol, and cocaine in particular, are used to mask and overcome painful feeling states and problems with self-esteem and dependency, it is important that these vulnerabilities be revealed gradually so that excessive defensiveness can be avoided, and members can develop an awareness of and a capacity to tolerate painful feeling states. While MDGT is supportive, it is designed ultimately to be expressive (i.e., uncovering and insight-oriented), but this is to be done in a manner and at a rate that preserves self-respect. The goal then is to maintain self-esteem and to try to focus gently and gradually on underlying painful affects and associated defenses rather than to insist that such defenses be surrendered (Khantzian, 1978).

A part of addicts' behavior is pleasure-seeking, but in a larger sense, beyond addiction, they are seeking through drugs an elusive psychological happiness that will erase or soothe their pain, and make life effortless and without suffering. As with psychotherapy in general, the goal of MDGT is in part, to have the addicts surrender this temporary and futile pursuit in favor of a genuine involvement in life, and to facilitate a maturing of the capacities for engagement with others, a less self-centered position, and an acceptance of the inevitable pain and genuine pleasures of reality.

CHAPTER VI

The Brass Heart:
Early Phases of the Group

MDGT is designed to be a time-limited group psychotherapeutic experience. Its twice per week, twenty-six week format places it in an intermediate range between short-term and long-term group psychotherapy. Depending on the setting, the processes and principles described here, with some modification, can and do apply as well to a more long-term format. However, unless specified otherwise, what follows is based on the assumption that MDGT is time limited to twenty-six weeks. Although this manual was devised for use with cocaine addicts, with slight modifications it can be easily adapted for use with substance abusers in general.

Most group therapists would agree that there is some degree of predictability, orderliness, and progression in the phases and development of a group. What follows should serve a group leader as a guide to help anticipate and identify characteristic qualities, processes, and events which develop in the life of an MDGT experience. The description of the group phases is based in part on an appreciation of the literature (see especially Gruen, 1977) and our own experiences in running psychodynamic psychotherapeutic groups. In what follows we will describe three group phases—a beginning phase, a middle phase, and an advanced/termination phase. There is no strict demarcation between the phases, as each group has a tendency to remain at and/or progress to a subsequent phase at varying rates.

In this rotating, open-group membership model, new participants are joining while others are completing their group tenure. There is therefore a moving back and forth between phases, which reflects the presence both of new and old members in the same groups. Themes of early recovery intertwine and resonate with the expressions of growing confidence and psychological maturation of the more senior members. While the phases thus remain fluid, the general tone and thrust of the group is largely set by the intermediate and senior members. For purposes of describing the phases we have divided the stages into three 17-session periods of time, further subdividing phase III (see Chapters 8 and 9) into three phases, "Unfinished Business" (Sessions 36–44), "Another Crisis" (Sessions 45–52), and "Nora's Story."

Beyond the specific guidelines provided in the early meetings in which the group leader takes the initiative and states the purpose, ground rules, and overall goals and philosophy of the program, he/she thereafter exercises a varying degree of initiative in subsequent meetings. Of course, as part of his/her modeling role, there is more need at first for the leader to foster interaction, with frequent reminders of the purpose and goals already stated. The group leader should over time also seek to balance a spontaneous development of the group interactions, with a more actively directed focus to assure that the affective, self-esteem, relationship, self-care, and character problems associated with their drug dependency are addressed.

Our assumption is that drug dependency is closely linked to self-governance problems, and more often than not, these difficulties spontaneously emerge over time. The group leader needs to use patience and judgment in deciding how active to be in drawing out and encouraging the development of the major themes/foci around these problems and the need to support, clarify (label, instruct, explain), confront, and interpret the bases of the interactions in the group. A central assumption is that what is helpful and healing is potentially available from the other members. A main responsibility of the group leader is to assess what is needed (e.g. support or interpretation), to facilitate and evoke the needed response from the members, and to provide it when the members are unable to or are slow in responding. Beyond insuring that the specified focus and content of MDGT are covered, the group leader, by example and modeling, must also help the group members keep in mind that they all share responsibility for developing optimal conditions for the work of the group—that is, maintaining an atmosphere of safety, comfort, and honesty, as well as a respectful attitude of speaking, listening, and support.

BEGINNING PHASE (SESSIONS 1–17)

Most individuals starting group struggle with how they will fit in. This concern is part of the self-consciousness of joining a group in which anxieties about exposure of self loom large. This is evident in the embarrassment and shame reactions, or exaggerated defensiveness so often seen in groups initially, and subsequently as deeper layers of the self are revealed and explored. The group leader should be sensitive to these reactions, especially early in the group history, and can be very helpful by indicating that such reactions are normal. This kind of sensitivity, which the group leader demonstrates and imparts, helps the members to deal with their concerns about belonging, acceptance, and fitting in, which are paramount early in the group, and persist more or less (for some more than others) throughout the group's life. Because of the newness of the experience and concerns about safety and security in this phase, discussion of topics and group interaction are often stereotypical and should be allowed for (i.e., not excessively challenged). Also, during this initial phase members search for norms as to what can be safely revealed and what the group will mean to them. Leo's self-consciousness in Vignette #2 is a good example of a patient's search for norms and for an acceptable topic for discussion early in a group's history. Leo's case also demonstrates how the leader can help members establish norms for safe self-revelation.

The wish to be liked and accepted in this phase significantly influences the type and quality of responses in the group interactions. Paradoxically, despite the wish for acceptance, even in this phase some members almost immediately invite rejection based on a negative self-image and characterological problems. Members in this phase are isolated from each other, hold back much, and concentrate on external events such as drugs and drug-related problems. They are either unable or unwilling to reveal their feelings and psychological suffering. Members in this phase fear disapproval, abandonment, and exclusion by the other members or the therapist, as well as fears of being considered pathological, crazy, or sick, and tend to see involvement in psychotherapy as confirmation of their fears about themselves and stereotypes about therapy.

Much of the anxiety and fear about starting group are beyond the members' awareness. The therapist's responsibility, as in individual psychotherapy, is to help people become aware of emotions, characteristic attitudes, and assumptions that operate automatically and, often as a consequence, deleteriously, in their lives, especially in symptomatic ways such as depending on drugs. Thus, the way these first-stage anxieties are managed is particularly important. The group leader attempts to gradually draw out members by helping them to identify their anxieties. Too much anxiety may lead to flight, and the absence or denial of anxiety may deprive a member of any impetus to master the challenge of opening up and joining the group. The group leader chooses his words carefully, especially early in the group, to protect members from attack, shame, or premature self-disclosure, such as of traumatic material. The objective is to evoke and support, not to provoke and offend. For example, in this phase of the group, the therapist would say something like, "It is uncomfortable and you are understandably nervous about joining a group and talking about yourselves publicly." This as opposed to, "It is terrifying to join a group and, given your druthers, you would prefer to isolate yourself." Although the latter statement may also be correct, it runs the risk of prematurely exposing a member's worst fears while demeaning him or her for lacking courage.

In some instances members resist acknowledging the real pain in their lives; in others they are not in touch with their feelings or have difficulty putting them into words. Especially early in group, such members should not be left to flounder for themselves or to withdraw. At first the group leader can be more active in drawing out and labeling reactions, but over time he/she can help members to continue to do it for each other by supporting or applauding it when it occurs spontaneously in the group, or by evoking it from another member who seems sensitive to this particular kind of problem or to a particular member. Accordingly, a therapist might say, "John, I think it is great that you could see Joe's sadness from his facial expression and the way he was talking; it helped Joe and the other members be more aware of their own feelings, and it helped Joe start to talk about what's really going on with him."

The leader is a powerful force in shaping the group culture, climate, and staying power, and in recognising members' sensitivities. The therapist can often gently put into words the fears that the member cannot or will not acknowledge or express. Beyond articulating an individual's fears or concerns, the leader can discuss such reactions in a way that invites a sharing of similar experiences and concerns from the other members. For example, the group leader might say something like, "Is Mary the only one who feels like a wallflower when she joins in with a new group of people?" That is, the group leader underscores the idea that people are not alone with their feelings of doubt, anxiety, estrangement, confusion, and embarrassment, and understands that the realization that others share these concerns is helpful. It is not too soon in this phase to articulate the theme, which needs constant rearticulation throughout the group's history, that "feelings are neither good nor bad, they just are." The leader also, for example, honestly acknowledges that "feelings that are painful might get worse before they get better, but staying and being with each other's feelings helps us to stay with our own distress better."

There is a growing recognition by the members, even in this phase, that problems are within oneself and not out there in the past, in others, or in the drug. However, as this happens the leader often becomes a target, for example, of anger because he/she is not continuing to set goals, not leading, or does not have all the answers. Being neither defensive, patronizing, nor indifferent (often not easy), the leader acknowledges the frustration, reality-tests extreme distortions, and facilitates interactions which help members to realize they can generate many of the explanations and answers among themselves. Sometimes this may occur by a simple response by the leader such as, "I don't recognize me," when a member articulates that the leader is too great a source of wisdom or a threat. The leader might add, "You must have your own special reasons for reacting to me that way, but let's see what others feel and think."

The group leader plays an important role in helping members appreciate that the frustration, fear, dependency, fight-flight, and other reactions that occur in and outside of group, which often cause problems, can conversely become opportunities in group for understanding and modifying their life problems. The leader can tactfully say the above and then wonder out loud about what the roots of group members' reactions might be. It is important in these beginning phases to reassure members that feelings and fears are a normal part of group work and not a sign of weakness or lack of worth, and that staying with and considering their own reactions is part of the work of the group. The constant observation of self and others produces a special pressure on members to be dissatisfied with old ways of acting and interacting.

The members then begin to move to a new middle phase where it is safer to disclose and share more about one's inner self, including more honest and open reactions about how one feels and thinks about oneself and others in the group. However, the group members and the leader constantly consolidate and hold themselves and each other to the important lessons learned in the beginning phase of group, namely, that sharing, exploration, and understanding occur in respectful, safe, friendly, and reasonably comfortable contexts—conditions that are everyone's responsibility.

As an example of the productive work of the MDGT group in its earliest phase we offer some of the powerful themes and images of the defended and wounded, yet still life-seeking, self that emerge, even during the staggering, immediate aftermath of severe drug dependency. In early MDGT groups one central theme that is articulated is the lifetime history of the attempt to harden oneself to feelings of vulnerability. In Session # 8, one of the members, Dan, describes once finding a brass heart in an antique shop, and how this seemed to capture for him all at once his yearning for intimacy, the cold, metallic defense against being injured or vulnerable, and the brazen, glittery surface that invites but does not yield. In a much earlier session, Dan had described himself as a crab who withdraws into his shell when he feels hurt.

Leo, a man in his late 40s, abandoned by his parents as a child, says he desires to be close to women, yet finds it less painful to relate to them only as though they were a "24-hour convenience store," rather than as people. He describes his many years of drug use as, in part, a controlled way of relating to others: "Once you let them in it's all over." He describes vividly how his adult life has been like living in a narrow alleyway, and how the effort to ward off the threat of pain from others keeps him trapped in this constricted space. These limitations are preferable to taking risks with others because the fear is greater than the desire, yet the longing for connection with others persists and is expressed even in the drug-taking itself.

The glittery, frenzied, thrilling, X-rated cocaine life appears to be the only antidote to the monotony of ordinary, everyday life as they experience it. The drugs seem to offer them an infusion of life in a safe, invulnerable way which avoids the loss of control they dread. The desire for a connection to life remains alive even though the attempts to satisfy this desire may be self-defeating, even life-threatening.

Even in this early group, members strikingly display characteristic themes and character structure, and deepen our understanding of the self-medication hypothesis. They describe forcefully how prior to using drugs their lives had become constricted and narrowed, and how they were estranged from others. The use of drugs was in part a way to find a safe, controlled place where life could come alive once more. Even though the venture miscarries and leads to an extreme loss of control, it is life-seeking. The MDGT group is a place to begin to reflect on these images of defense and desire, and to begin to understand the shared patterns that these images and stories evoke.

MIDDLE PHASE (SESSIONS 18–34)

The middle phase is ushered in as members feel increasingly involved and connected to the group as a whole and begin to experience special attachments to one another. In this phase the members often begin to evoke special and often troubling feelings and perceptions about self and others. As we will see subsequently crises concerning continued attendance, absences, and/or drug use often occur at these times. Skillful management of these crises can enhance rather than jeopardize the cohesiveness of the group.

The lessons gained in the previous phase of acceptance and support for expressing uncomfortable reactions lead to members assuming an increasingly active and reflective role, but the group leader remains alert for subtle and inadvertent lapses in sensitivity when members demean, derogate, or overlook troublesome verbal and non-verbal communications about self and others. For example, a member, Bill, may betray impatience toward another member, Jane, which while partly deserved by Jane, also betrays unique and intemperate qualities in Bill. The group leader might say, "Bill, you seemed impatient when Jane told the story of how worried she was about her cat who was sick. I/we know Jane can overreact, making it hard for herself and others, but I wonder if you can see that you react very strongly yourself, perhaps more strongly than others—and I wonder if it isn't related to your usual problem when people emote too much. Maybe Jane and you can benefit if you and the group try to figure out together what happens inside each of you and between you." With this kind of observation the group members draw on their inside and outside of group knowledge of each other to help both Bill and Jane observe and modify their characteristic behaviors and ways of responding to each other and other members. As we can see, in this stage more habitual, characterological (i.e. characteristic) ways of interacting are evident, and individuals find their own unique ways for positioning themselves in the group. The members progressively see themselves during this phase as more worthy of attention and more self-accepting as they internalize the accepting, supportive attitude of the group leader and other members. In this period there is greater emphasis on personality dynamics, character structure, and an increased sense of self-efficacy and autonomy. Members take pleasure in offering help to other members and there is a marked loosening of defenses, with self-protection giving way to self-expression.

It is also during this phase that the group leader encourages group members to elaborate and amplify on experiences inside and outside group which typify the feeling, self-esteem, relationship, self-care, and character problems that lead to drug dependency and other self-defeating solutions to problems in living.

GROUP VIGNETTE #4

Self-expression versus Self-protection

The following vignette provides an example of an MDGT group in the middle phase. In this hour we key on Ralph, a 31-year-old man embarking on a new career, and Paul, a 21-year-old macho man who, at the time of this meeting, have been in group for approximately 16 weeks (32 group sessions). Although Paul has tended to be flamboyant and colorful, he has periodically demonstrated touching sensitivity to others' distress and has also manifested a growing candor about himself. In this hour both men reveal an expanding capacity to express their feelings about themselves and their lifestyles, and are learning to endure and enjoy life without drugs. This meeting also demonstrates how a successful group experience helps individuals to loosen up their defenses, while at the same time helping to increase their awareness of how characteristic (or characterologic) defenses operate to protect against the threat of unwanted feelings and difficult relationships. In this meeting it is evident that money, relationships (especially sexuality), and drugs may serve to maintain an inflated sense of self when in fact a more hidden, unsure, and disabled self lurks and needs to surface for purposes of acceptance, nurturance, care, and growth. This meeting begins with Paul seizing the lead after a preliminary period of playful banter and chit chat.

PAUL: I used to pimp, sell drugs, get busted. I was never convicted. I'm the type of guy you want to keep away from your daughters. I was a sickness trying to love.

LEADER: You have a terminal illness then, because you will never get over it now, and you can never go back to the tough and cold person you were.

PAUL: All my women are lovely. I date beautiful women but everything around me seems to be falling apart. But I'm in a good mood. I'm finding out about the way people really are and the way women are. I put them on the pedestal, but the bitches are playing me for my friends. I wouldn't expect women to act the way I acted.

LEADER: Feeling love for someone is a weakness?

PAUL: That's the truth. It's a weakness. I went through changes behind my feelings. I had to go and talk in groups. I should just fuck around and have fun, and not fall in love. There's no in between for me. I'm being nice, and I'm not in control of what's going on.

LEADER: You mean nice like your mother was, and people take advantage of that.

PAUL: Before I never trusted any bitch, anyone. I still got plenty of women...many of them use drugs...in various stages of use and abuse.

LEADER: With cocaine you had a lot of power over women?

PAUL: But I still got power, and they still get hooked on Paul now, and there's no detox from Paul! I'm good at meeting bitches, but not at love.

LEADER: Love causes you pain.

PAUL: I always felt I was missing something. I'm not good at love.

LEADER: Just after you stopped drugs you had two experiences with women and you were vulnerable and they didn't work out. So now you see your only option as going back to being the tough guy. We have other experts here on relationships and love. It's hard to find out what reality is like, what women are like…and regrets over what you did or didn't do.

PAUL: I always wanted to be a computer programmer. While on drugs I could accomplish nothing. Now I have an opportunity…now that I am not addicted anymore.

LEADER: Is what you are talking about now something that might make you use drugs? Another rejection from someone you really like or a blow to your self-esteem in the future?

PAUL: Nothing can make me slip…unless I forget where I came from and what I went through.

LEADER: You're going somewhere now with your life, in the right direction, working, school, ambition….

PAUL: I'm glad you have more faith in my abilities than I do.

Although in his language and manner Paul still exhibits aspects of his previous aggressive, dominant, and macho style, it is also clear that he is changing. The exchange between the leader and Paul clicks away, is engaging, mildly confrontative yet supportive, and mutually respectful.

The group and the leader next shift to Ralph, who's background is different, but whose struggles and problematic issues are shared by Paul and others in the group. This central theme of relationships and compulsive drug use continues.

RALPH: It's the first time in my life that I haven't had a girlfriend or wife. It's weird. I used to live in three apartments at once, then I moved in with a girl to get away from what was going on in the other places.

LEADER: A high octane life since you were a kid?

RALPH: I've had no drink in ten weeks, and no coke in five months. I was married for ten years and I can't remember anything about it. This other woman, Barbara, was my coke partner. It played on my mind something terrible. I got a Dear John from her in jail. She lives nearby, and her husband is a nut. He was following me around. He's in A.A. I didn't even know she was married the first year I lived with her, but I knew she had kids. He turned me into the police for coke. He used to sneak around my house and he had people following me. I was riding around with a gun myself, and I'm lucky I didn't shoot someone. She got into trouble with prescriptions. She owed Colombians some money. The cops caught me at my house. I still miss her a lot, and I don't know whether I hate her or love her. Sexually she was incredible. I cashed a check for seventeen grand on a Friday night and by next Thursday we were broke.

LEADER: Was it all so painful you wanted to blot it out?

RALPH: I was never faithful to my first wife…we were only like friends… we had to get married.

LEADER: Now it's a lonely time for you?

RALPH: I never took women or feelings seriously. I am a workaholic, I always was. Money is important to me. (Ralph uses money as a self-object, like Paul uses women, in order to shore up a fragile sense of self).

LEADER: You tell it all and you make it funny, yet the story is painful— years of lovelessness and pain and being out of control.

RALPH: Yes, but I had five years of being clean in upstate New York when I was teaching.

LEADER: How was that? Clean for years when you were teaching, and teaching is not a high paying job for a moneyman. What was the relationship between working and staying clean?

RALPH: The kids liked me. I fought administration policies about homework, and I was like the pied piper. I enjoyed teaching and coaching—soccer, basketball, softball. My team was county champs. I always coached, and I never had a coke problem. But I always worried about it. We had a baseball team that was so good. I taught them how to bunt and field. We beat teams 50-2. I enjoyed it...a little shithole town in New York State. The town threw us a parade when we won the county champs. It was the best feeling in my life.

LEADER: How did you end up in a small town?

RALPH: I did everything there. I have eight years of a suspended sentence now. I only had to do forty-nine days. I could've got "not guilty" if I hadn't been so fucked up on drugs.

LEADER: You led a wild life, family all high, then you sober up and take a town by storm and make a tremendous impact, like the Music Man. Then you stopped and went back to a drug life.

RALPH: I was a fireman, and head of the local teachers' association...no deceits or lies then...I was smarter than anyone in the town...but then my ex-wife's mother got sick. We had to go take care of her...we were going to get the house later, but we didn't...that was the end of my marriage.

LEADER: You were it in the town. Was it dull for you...the church socials...the small town life?

RALPH: Apparently not...I loved the fire department, civic committees, and all that. I took kids camping, and I was always busy. Starkville! I bought softball jerseys for the whole team at work, just like I buy breakfast now for my whole staff now every morning.

LEADER: They must have a statue of you in that town. Ralph Daman Day...Damansville.

RALPH: They loved me for all I did there, and the causes I fought for them (like fighting with police but in a productive way)...people there were like sheep. I fought hard for them and stood up to outsiders who bullied them.

LEADER: It sounds like you have some remarkable abilities.

RALPH: I did so much, I put everything into it. The whole town knew me and liked me...it was great.

LEADER: The Music Man, The Human Tornado, comes to Damansville.

RALPH: I shouldn't have talked so much tonight.

LEADER: We're really upset you talked so much.

RALPH: It was so nice in here tonight.

LEADER: It sounds like who you are and what you can do you can do anywhere when your energy and dedication have direction.

As with Paul, this has been a meeting where the leader and Ralph make good contact with each other and as they speak to each other, they do so in a way from which others can benefit. Because it is uncharacteristic for this group to be limited to interactions with one or two members, Ralph feels self-conscious about monopolizing the group. However, the acceptability and utility of this kind of interaction is evident from the spontaneity of the exchange and the sense of benefit and appreciation that Paul and Ralph display and express. In the early phase of the group this is important because although there is a legitimate concern about "equal time," it is also appropriate on certain occasions that "fair shares" (Balint, 1972) are not necessarily measured by temporal considerations alone.

The work of the previous 34 meetings has fostered increasing openness, sharing, and attachment. Despite tensions and discomforts around certain issues and even the crises that emerged as the group developed, this group has come a considerable way. From being a collection of individuals brought together by their common problem with cocaine, they have become a cohesive unit, with a sense of themselves as a group and as individuals who share other common ground beyond addiction. Perhaps more than at any other time in their lives, they have sustained and been sustained in an extraordinary human context. They have learned new ways of seeing themselves and others, and about private and personal matters that have been a source of pain, confusion, embarrassment, shame, loneliness, and need. They have discovered a more effective, validating, and reassuring way to deal with their difficulties, which have been and might otherwise remain painfully internalized and repetitiously perpetuated through action and self-defeating attachments and behavior.

With this background the final phase, including termination, permits increased self-disclosure and sharing of feelings, more genuine interactions, and a growing awareness on the part of the members of their ability to cope. Members take more responsibility for the feelings they experience and evoke and accept the individuality of others in the group (including the leader). They also feel (more or less) increasing independence from the therapist as they internalize the leader's and members' therapeutic attitudes toward self.

Termination, or more simply put, saying good-bye to each other, extends over this period. Members express appropriate feelings of happiness and even enthusiasm for knowing each other and growing together, as well as sadness for losing the group and the special relationships it has provided. Members reminisce, recapitulate, and continue to work over and work through the unique ways their particular vulnerabilities have played themselves out. There is a growing respect as well for the unique qualities and strengths they have come to appreciate in themselves and others in the group. Special reactions toward the leader and reciprocal feedback from the leader often amplify how vulnerabilities have been worked out and the special positive qualities of each member have been acknowledged, consolidated, and enjoyed.

CHAPTER VII

Unfinished Business: The Group in Crisis

While this group has been successful through its early phase in establishing cohesiveness, having no dropouts, nor any reported cocaine or illicit drug use, the work is far from done. There remains, in the words of one of the members, much "unfinished business."

This reference to "unfinished business" means that the group members are starting to see how they manage their lives and how they regard the world and themselves; they are starting to understand the self-regulating functions mediated by cocaine. "Unfinished business" means that as character problems emerge in the group, members can begin to explore options and alternatives to these characteristic, maladaptive ways of seeing self, others, and reality. At this point they begin to see that the future is open to the extent that they have choices and can do things differently—whether interacting with others, managing feelings, or in the way they care for and regard themselves. What had been automatic about addiction and character is now open to reflection and review.

We will focus in this chapter on the group in crisis. This is a critical issue at all stages of the MDGT group. It is the primary task of the leader to handle as well as he or she can the multilayered dimensions of any group crisis in order to preserve the group's existence and to further its progress. The work of the group at all phases hinges on an acceptable resolution of crisis.

We focus here, for instructional purposes, on the crises of poor attendance and the threat of premature termination by several group members. Such developments are typical of group crises but they may take many forms, such as the use of drugs or alcohol by members, the inability to regulate affect storms in group, the scapegoating of a group member, failures in the management of cravings, problems caused by extra-group contact between members, narcissistic crises, and issues external to the group that place a member or members in personal crisis. Here we will look primarily on the group in crisis around a premature termination in order to show how any crisis, managed adequately, often furthers group development and successful treatment outcome.

PSYCHOLOGICAL RELAPSE

No matter how well the group has fared in terms of abstinence, cohesiveness, increased self-awareness, and self-exoneration, it is still at grave risk of psychological relapses that are more endangering than symptomatic drug relapses. Just as group members at all times remain at high risk for drug relapse, so too the group is always at risk of fragmentation, poor intragroup relations, affect intolerance, and Wall Street-like crashes of self-esteem.

The situation may appear rosy as members speak glowingly of success in their life and pleasure in the group, but this can rapidly unravel. Groups, in all phases of their development, may be conceived as opportunities for either psychological relapse or psychological recovery of both the individual members and the group. It is critical that the leader be ever-vigilant in spotting and managing these crises, and when possible using them as an opportunity for members to gain increased insight into the areas of psychological functioning and character structure which this manual emphasizes throughout.

The MDGT group can lead to an increased sense of self-efficacy, enhanced self-esteem, improved interpersonal relations, more positive self-care, increased tolerance of painful affect states, and a growing capacity to come to grips with life on a more realistic psychological terrain. As treatment progresses, members ideally will gain a better knowledge of their character structure, a stronger sense of how they have managed in the past to deal with these central issues, and a greater flexibility in their responses to life. The maladaptive but ego-syntonic aspects of psychological functioning that to date have caused so much suffering may become increasingly ego-alien. The member learns that there are other solutions to his or her problems, or as Bibring (1954) writes:

> By seeing his difficulties more clearly and in a more objective, realistic perspective he is no longer overwhelmed or frightened by them; he is less identified with them; no longer takes them for granted, nor does he consider them as constitutional parts of personality. (p. 757)

The work of the MDGT group can be conceptualized as a model of psychological relapse prevention. It aims to help the patient find a solution to the problem of the self without drugs or an automatic return to action, and to the psychological extremism of uncontrollable anger, impulsivity, painful emptiness, all-or-nothing responses, or self-abdication when difficult times arise. Group members slowly realize that the search—through drugs, food, another person, money, or sex—for external and magical solutions to the problem of the self does not yield a long-lasting resolution. Insofar as drug use is a flight from and attempt to artificially enhance oneself, then the MDGT group is the road back to oneself, to an acknowledgment of one's real hurts and life conflicts.

The group would for the most part rather talk about drinking, drugs, attendance, conflict, or war stories, in other words, anything other than what calls out always as central: the pain and suffering that are uniquely one's own. Group members are challenged to see that they are people who have settled on a powerful chemical solution to their conflicts that magically takes away depression, makes the frightened brave, the shy confident, the fragmented whole, the grieving forgetful, and the failed successful.

Every MDGT group should be seen by the leader as an opportunity for psychological relapse or psychological recovery. It is never a question of members simply getting better or of problems receding into the distance. The group's being in crisis is the norm, and its resolution is the crux of the work of the group. The earlier that members can begin to reflect on this notion, the greater the chance to be able to work through more painful and dangerous crises as they appear during the life of the group. The supportive–expressive style of the MDGT leader uses the crisis as an opportunity to provide an increased awareness and a greater sense of choice concerning how conflict and ambivalence are managed both in group and in life.

THE COMMON GROUND AND THE MIDDLE GROUND

Addictions and obsessions in the lives of group members reflect a tendency toward psychological extremism and intolerance of ambivalence. Such extremism and inability to tolerate ambivalence give rise to both the crisis and the inability to resolve it constructively. It is easier to quit, storm out, get high, sulk, and act out than to understand what is going on. The member or the group in crisis will invariably manifest this trend. Life, oneself, and others in the group are idealized or devalued. The middle ground is not a familiar or sought after place for them. They tend to romanticize and glorify extreme positions, though this leads again and again to a sad and vicious adaptation to life, leaving them in debt, often in physical jeopardy, and at times unable to sustain relationships or work. For example, one group member, in a discussion about sex and recovery, described himself as a "sex animal" who participated frequently in orgiastic encounters. He could not imagine sex without drugs, yet he saw his recovery as necessitating his finding a "church-going woman" to live with in a house with a white picket fence. He saw the life of recovery as one without real pleasure, as if the price of ordinary life were one of unremitting drudgery and joyless obligation. These contrasting images served as common ground for the group discussion, and evoked a surprising degree of unanimity around these extremely polarized and stereotyped beliefs.

Albeit self-defeating, this way of looking at things is ego-syntonic, comfortable, and automatic. The work of the leader is to focus on this extremist tendency, to survey the middle ground in members' lives and in the life of the group, and to contrast the ordinary aspects and demands of life with the extraordinary experiences sought through drugs or other means. Frequently, the work of the group is to better understand how one can find genuine pleasure and satisfaction in ordinary life.

When one member places the group in crisis, it is also an opportunity for the leader to help all the members find the common ground where the most productive work gets done. While the group members initially came together around their common problem of drug dependence, the leader's aim is to move the group to other sources of commonality: psychological and life experiences in the four dimensions MDGT emphasizes. This new common ground is an opportunity for insight into oneself and connection with others.

We will see in the following transcripts how the seemingly central and personal issue of attendance fast becomes peripheral as the group explores various conflicts such as vulnerability, dysfunctional patterns of self-care, and core relationship themes. The crisis often begins as an eroding or volatile issue but can lead to a common ground, and if successfully managed, to an increased sense of regard for self and others, and a growing, even if reluctant, appreciation for less extremist solutions to problems.

In our experience, some of the important ingredients in this process include the ongoing affectionate banter, teasing, play, and humor that develops among the members during the life of the group. Grunebaum and Solomon (1980, 1982, 1987) have underscored the developmental importance of peers and how the elements of play and esteem of others that evolve in group therapy can compensate for previously unsuccessful peer relationships, and help to develop and maintain improved self-esteem.

The problems of the early phase of the group are different in quality, but not in kind, from the crises that emerge in later phases of the group. For example, the central issues of attendance and premature termination are present from the very start. It is more helpful conceptually to see the group in its temporal entirety, and not as disconnected, separate series of events. The character dynamics of the members, and the nature of the transference are present from first to last. The outcome is uncertain, and can turn sour if the group is unable to deal effectively with a crisis as it arises.

In this final phase of the group we see refrains and variations of crises and character patterns that are familiar to us from the early groups, yet they are different here in that they now come into high relief, when the group knows each other well, is cohesive, and has had a period of drug-free life behind them.

THE GROUP ON THE EDGE OF DISSOLUTION

The first group we will examine in this phase is at Session #39. This group is in crisis around the issues of lapses in attendance, ambivalence regarding continuation of treatment, and the possibility of premature termination by several members. An analysis of this group meeting is illustrative of many of the themes and techniques applicable to any MDGT group at any phase.

The road to psychological recovery depends on continuing in the group. The group is in danger of fragmentation, and it is not clear that the group will weather this threat or that the forces favoring recovery and continuation will win out over those of withdrawal, dissolution, and relapse.

GROUP VIGNETTE #5

At this group meeting all members are present for the first time in several weeks. Morgan has missed the previous three meetings, and was very angry when last seen. Al has expressed to his individual counselor his wish to leave group because of problems at school. Nora has yet to make any real connection to the group, and is often vocal about her dissatisfaction with the group's direction and focus. Matt has vacillated about being in the group since his first meeting. Several new members are present and their continuation in the group crucially depends on how this problem is handled. The group of ten people is now at risk of losing half or more of it members.

We see here the continued use of externalization as a central defense in regard to both group dynamics and the issue of members' drug use. It is disconcerting to reflect on oneself or to share one's suffering with the group, and so now, where originally members had come to group with the expectation of getting better in some passive, magical way, the group itself has become the problem, summoning up ancient, repetitious characterological patterns. This mid-phase group has an intensity that allows for increased disclosure, greater affect, heightened self-reflection, and for the bearing of ambivalent feelings concerning self and others.

The characteristic way of managing difficult conflict situations for these group members in the past has been to take flight and quit what they started. This is the psychological relapse that may be averted by clarification when it arises. By entertaining the option of dropping out, group members again confirm their old view of self as failed and deficient, and the world as disappointing. Remaining in the group goes against the characterologic grain, and it is against this grain that the therapist often focuses his or her work, pointing out the pattern of fear, flight, and failure, and presenting the option of remaining instead of running.

When the leader first becomes aware of the crisis of a member or of the group, it must be the main order of business when the group convenes. At times the leader may be empathic and supportive, while at other times a more direct, confrontational, though tactful, approach is required. The leader's objective is to use this current crisis as an opportunity for the group to move to some common ground, to explore the middle ground, to avoid irreparable fragmentation, and to lead to an increased self-awareness by all group members, no matter how limited or broad this crisis may be.

Session #39

As the group assembles tonight the usual friendly banter fills the room. Instead of his normally letting it move on to a topic of common interest, the leader interrupts to address the current problem of attendance.

LEADER: There are some important things going on in the group we need to discuss. One is attendance. Matt and Al missed last Thursday, and Nora missed last week. I wonder what's going on.

MORGAN: I was exhausted last Thursday.

NORA: I worked overtime everyday, went to school every night, was tired, and went home.

AL: I don't have any excuses. I missed two Thursdays in a row. I didn't call. Coming here interferes with my thing at school, and with other growth. Part of the problem with drugs is that they interfered with my growth but I always made it to lectures even when I was high. I'm in school for learning, and now this program interferes with that growth, and the reason I have any problem at all is that I'm not confident I can say "fuck this program" and forget about drugs. Drugs are still an issue and a problem that needs to be dealt with, but it seems a little regressive to remain in that drug problem, personal therapy, or other programs. So what's more important, going to these lectures and learning in school, or coming to these meetings? Except for a few meetings they haven't been amazing, haven't been the kind of meetings I feel I absolutely can't miss.

MATT: I'm new in this but I'm speaking for me, I was told that I had to make a commitment and that attendance is mandatory. I feel the same way as you, and don't get anything out of it sometimes, but I feel as a group, if a commitment is not made by each and every individual here it's going to affect the group. If it's okay for everyone to do it, then we'll all be missing. If this meeting is for recovery and you're not putting that first, then go do what you have to do, if you don't think this is important. I gotta keep my recovery first. I don't want to get high again, and I know if I don't come I'll get high again. I'd rather be working sometimes, and I miss the money I could make, but I have to come here.

AL: I agree. I have to decide whether to stay in the group. I have to think about the commitment to the program and to myself, and the value of that commitment in comparison to other things. Certainly it's crucial not to use drugs, but I have doubts as to whether I need meetings to stay off drugs. I need something to force me to continually acknowledge that I have this problem.

LEADER: (*returning to Al's statement*) I am interested in what this "amazing" means. What makes something amazing for you, and why that is important to you?

The leader responds to this devaluing comment since the group did not. Such comments are as frequent but in ways more dangerous and damaging than idealizing statements. They reflect the core narcissistic characterologic issues the group must grapple with at all phases. By asking the group member to clarify what he means the leader hopes to bring the automatic devaluing process into the awareness of the member and the group in order to move away from the manifest issue of staying or leaving, and toward the more central issues of characterologic patterns and choice. Implicit in Al's quest of the "amazing" is the common misconception of psychotherapy as a dramatic, intensely cathartic, and magical resolution for all psychological ailments. This view of psychotherapy implies a passive, mechanical model of change in which the individual waits for something to be done to him or her, or as an uncovering of some ancient traumatic event that will explain all difficulties.

AL: I don't know. I just don't feel too jeopardized by drugs now.

Over and over again the members focus on drug use as a resistance to self-reflection. Whenever this comes up the leader needs to reframe and restate the focus—to see how drug use fits into one's life, and the many meanings drugs have for the person in regard to the central MDGT issues.

LEADER: I don't see this group as dealing primarily with drugs. Over time you've spoken of drugs, how you see the world, your family, and others at work and here. You told us you felt no connection here. Even when the group was teasing you, you spoke of having no feelings and that it didn't phase you. I'd be hurt. To me a group is what you bring to it. Amazing groups, like amazing days, are unusual. Last week with Leo was an amazing group when he told us stories of psychosis, despair, and recovery.

MATT: I got a lot out of that when he shared with us, about where drugs can bring you.

LEADER: Leo gave us that gift. It's what people bring to it. You don't see yourself in that league of suffering, and you wonder how much drugs are a problem for you. You get lost in whether it is a disease or not. It's your experience of it that is important. This is not a show where something happens that you watch. If someone comes with what's real for them now then something is going to happen. I think you have a lot to bring to the group and get from the group. It's up to you.

AL: I have to travel 2 hours from Amherst.

LEADER: You made a commitment to come no matter what. I wonder if school is the issue. Let's imagine there is no conflict with school, what then?

AL: It's only school. Lectures at school are amazing. It's true I have much more difficulty in putting effort into this group than I do into school.

LEO: What do you want to do, Al?

AL: I want to quit and go to school.

LEO: Why did you come tonight?

AL: Because I am afraid to quit. This group somehow helps me fight drugs. I still think about drugs, and have an interest in them, and that scares me.

MORGAN: A commitment is a commitment. Paul doesn't fucking want to be here but he comes. I honestly feel, you can jump on it if you want, but we put too much fucking energy on whether people are here or not. We recover in the context of having a life and if he can only make it once a week, I'd rather have him here once than not be here at all, and you're pushing him out, to make a choice.

LEADER: I didn't say that. I like what you're saying, though.

MORGAN: The fact of the matter is we have so many other important things to talk about instead of attendance. It sounds like grade school. It does. Who's here are the people who want to be here. I really resent us spending a half hour of our time on this.

(Attendance and continuation in group are problems for Morgan and the group now. He has been drinking lately. He has not mentioned this in group, but told his individual counselor).

MATT: It seems to me that Al is still questioning whether he is an addict or not.

MORGAN: I think that we have so many other things to talk of. The issue of attendance has nothing to do with recovery.

LEO: I think it does.

MATT: Let's hear from others who haven't spoke, and let the majority rule.

LEADER: Let's not rush to vote.

LEO: I've broken a lot of commitments in my life. They asked me to make a commitment here. It is important. Breaking commitments and *leaving unfinished business* is the way we used to live. It bothers me as a group member. When somebody is missing, something is missing. If you are not there you are severely missed and I'm serious. Your input is missed. There's a lot we get from each other. It's a commitment not just to yourself but to this group that has to be fulfilled. You gave your word. I don't think anyone should be dropped off.

DAN: There were many times when I was tired and did not want to come, but the cohesiveness of the group suffers when we don't come on a regular basis. I missed you last week when you weren't here.

RALPH: I would always make it here. I made a commitment. I can't picture what would happen in my life to make me not come here. Tuesday and Thursday for six months I'll be here no matter if anyone's here. It's weird for me here . It's like real people. It's like real stuff here, not slogans like N.A. meetings. I do not socialize at all other than here. I go to work, meetings, or here, nothing else. It's all so new to me.

NORA: Things happen, commitment or no commitment. You have to do what you have to do.

RALPH: Every time someone does not come I think they went out and got high. I saw so many people drop out of N.A. Here in this small group you really know who's not here.

LEO: If someone is not here my first reaction is to think the worst.

AL: This is why I have such a problem. I think this is good and valuable time here. If I thought this group not worthwhile, or too dogmatic, or not a good idea, then this would not be a difficult decision. For me my profession comes before anything else. It comes before recovery. My other commitment is to my education.

These interactions among the group members about Al's attitudes toward group commitment offer a powerful example of how the members, with helpful initiative from the leader, can mobilize concern for both group viability and the well-being of one of its members. To the extent that these responses are forthcoming from the members, the leader can listen and observe empathically. To the extent that the responses are not forthcoming or are met with heightened resistance which fosters impatience or withdrawal by the members, then the leader may have to intercede with a member such as Al, who, despite the eloquent pleas of his peers, characteristically places his priorities apart from the group and threatens its cohesiveness and continuity. In this case the group's support and concern create the ground for the leader to more actively confront Al's resistances, and as they emerge, the resistances of other reluctant members.

LEADER: How about your commitment, Al? What is the group to each of you? Why is it that no one in this group has gotten high? How come? Why is this group doing so well? What is the group to you, apart from the drug question?

AL: I'm just here for drugs. I don't respond well to groups and I don't like it all that much.

LEADER: What don't you like?

AL: I don't like the lack of focus. Issues that need real work can't be worked through in depth here.

LEADER: How is it, that if you have something important to discuss you feel you can't even bring it up here?

AL: I just feel that way. I couldn't even tell you if you said "What are your problems?" what my problems are. I know there are problems. Discovering what those problems are takes a lot of time and effort therapeutically speaking and there is not enough time in one hour. It wouldn't be fair to the others. Groups are most suited for crisis issues where you can say clearly what the problem is.

LEADER: If one of the problems I have in my life is with other people it becomes more apparent in a group than alone, seeing it in action, live and on stage, like the problem you mentioned of feeling special.

AL: I have been able to be more receptive to things outside myself from coming here.

NORA: You mean you're not so self-centered! (*Group laughs*)

AL: I've learned there are things about this world I don't know, and I've become more able to accept that instead of closing myself into a nice little unit.

LEADER: Like a cocoon. In some ways the group has helped you let the world in.

AL: The hardest part to leave is this thing I've just learned or discovered, and it needs work, maintenance. It's a place to realize there are other people and other points of view.

LEADER: It's not just other people, it's these people.

AL: At school when I argue I need to win. Here people are equal. This is a new experience for me.

Here Al's character style and way of relating to others emerge vividly and are challenged. Insight is not the sole province of the leader. Al and the other members offer ideas and images related to the narcissistic, position and the isolation it brings.

MORGAN: If he makes a decision are we going to vote him out of the group? If the group said they wanted you to come even if it could only be once a week, you wouldn't come?

AL: I wouldn't expect that to happen, but it'd be nice.

MORGAN: I feel you feel pressured to make an either–or decision. The group has changed since it began. People are working now, some of us were out of work then. That was an easy decision to make when we were not working and addicted.

LEO: That's not true. I was going to court, had a heavy jones, and an infection in my arm. We were all in very serious trouble!

DAN: Things are a lot easier for me now than when I first came into this group. There was a lot more turmoil in my life and in myself. Now I'm working harder but there's a lot less turmoil.

LEADER: We're not kicking anyone out or voting. Just talking.

MORGAN: I don't think it's going to be too long before I'm in the same position as Al.

MATT: I hope each person is responsible enough to make his or her own decision.

LEADER: The most interesting part is your talk about the group, Al.

MORGAN: I want this fucking issue resolved. I still feel weak.

LEADER: These people brought the world to you. Not just that someone is not here, but that person is not here, and missing that person. You make it sound like people in general made you more aware of the world, and not these specific people. What would it be like leaving people you've known for so long?

AL: There's nobody in this group that's so dynamic that they cut through something I had. I allowed it to happen. I might pick Leo as the one example of someone who is so dynamic.

NORA: Can I say something? It's this conversation that makes it very hard for me to continue to make a commitment to this group. Jesus Christ! This is boring the fuck out of me. I don't believe I'm sitting here listening to this. I feel like this a lot of times when I come in here. We thrash it over too much. I feel like I want to scream. This is not worth my time or energy talking about absenteeism for a fucking hour when there's other things I'd rather be doing. It's beginning to be a waste of my time and effort to come here for this bullshit.

AL: I am the one who is talking , and I like talking, and it's my problem.

LEADER: : I'm very interested in whether you are going to stay in the group.

DAN: I don't think the real issue is absenteeism. I think the real issue is commitment. My life is a history of broken commitments and for me this program is important and I'm keeping my word. I've broken my word so many times, it's important to me just to keep it this once.

MATT: Well said. I feel the same way. My whole life has been a series of broken promises. The only things I've ever finished in my life are two drug rehabs. That's pretty sad. This is the first thing positive I've ever done in my life.

MORGAN: I don't need this shit. I'm getting real fucking mad. I've got to worry about coming here, and I got to deal with this shit. It really pisses me off. Kick me out or tell me I can stay, or let me fucking go! We're going around in fucking circles. It's bullshit, man! I don't want to fucking quit. I need this group.

Here Morgan sets up others as controlling his life, and then fights them angrily. While he recognizes his ambivalence, he externalizes the choice about staying or leaving, and looks to the leader or the group to resolve his problem.

LEADER: I didn't even know you were thinking of quitting.

MORGAN: I feel I got two fucking options. I can come here twice a week or I can leave.

LEO: I didn't hear anyone else say that.

LEADER: I didn't know this was an issue.

MORGAN: I got to go out of town for six weeks

LEADER: You mentioned once you might have to miss some meetings, but you haven't spoken of it with us since.

NORA: So he misses a couple of nights because of his job, that's cool.

LEADER: Al is talking about something else, about quitting the group. His ambivalence is about the group itself. The group hasn't said anything to you.

RALPH: I don't think it's as important what we're talking about so much as the ways of looking at the problem, whatever it is. This is really amazing to me. I'm so used to singular, either—or thinking, and always trying to manipulate others to come around to my way. I'm really awestruck at what's happening here tonight. I'm flabbergasted!

LEADER: You're angry in a way you're not usually, Morgan.

MATT: I want you in the group. I get a lot out of what you have to say. I don't want you to leave.

MORGAN: I didn't know this was going to come up.

RALPH: If this were chemotherapy instead of psychotherapy you'd be here. Would you say, "No chemo for me this week. I'm tired. I've got to go to a lecture"?

LEADER: We were talking about Al and you blow into a rage about this issue and want an immediate decision. I wonder how that works. Is it just here, just now, that this happens?

MORGAN: I need this program.

LEO: I'd like to work out a solution.

AL: It's not just the Thursday lectures. I can't afford five hours to do this every week.

NORA: You keep doing that intellectualizing shit.

LEADER: I don't want you to leave the group. I hope you'll continue.

LEO: We need to work out a solution. This thing is tearing at both of you inside.

LEADER: Al, I'm glad you brought this up tonight. I like what Dan said about cohesiveness. This is a good group. We have a lot of unfinished business, as Leo said before, and we'll get back to it at the next meeting.

At group's end the crisis is unresolved. Morgan is angry. Matt is still debating whether to continue. The new members are confused about their recent commitment to the rules of the group in light of the older members' doubts. Al still wants to leave, and Nora would likely be not far behind him. The group was successful in not making a premature decision based on external factors, and in learning how to discuss and bear the tension of conflicts and painful affects without taking flight.

An important common ground theme that takes shape in the hour is that of unfinished business, broken promises, and patterns of quitting. The group will return to this theme in the following hours, and it will be an important ingredient in their final decision to stay or go, helping to shape the direction and mood of the group over the next few months.

CHAPTER VIII

Becoming Vulnerable: Crisis Resolution

At the meeting following the discussion of "unfinished business," Morgan and Al were noticeably absent. It was a good group with a sharp reduction in tension. The group appeared unconcerned about the missing members. At this session, #41, all members were present for what became a turning-point session. Four or more members still remained at risk for termination, and Al informed the leader before group that he had decided to terminate. This session illustrates the potency of the group to reach and soften, if only for a time, the core vulnerability and narcissistic character structure of Al, who to date never made a real connection with the group.

GROUP VIGNETTE #6: (NARCISSISTIC VULNERABILITY)

Session #41

The group begins with Morgan angrily raising his hand to be called on.

LEADER: We have to raise our hands to speak here?

MORGAN: I'm really pissed off at this group, and at you. I very dogmatically asked for an answer a week ago. I didn't get it. And you very definitely changed the conversation at the time I asked you last week. I had to make a decision as to what I was going to do, about my work project that means a whole hell of a lot to me. And I didn't get an answer and I had to make a decision on what I thought was incomplete information, and I had to give up this project of mine. I did not get an answer from my group.

MATT: First of all you made your decision and now you just have to live with it. The way it seemed to me it was left last week was that you were real angry. The issue was not about you. It was about Al. You kind of jumped in and got real angry, like we were forcing you to make a choice, and that never came across to me. The way the group put it was if there were situations that had to be dealt with at work we could work around it.

MORGAN: I didn't get that at all, man. I was asking for an answer. I took it as, "No, Morgan! If you're going to miss all the Thursdays you're out of the group. " I told the group I had business.

LEADER: Last Thursday you had out-of-town business?

MORGAN: No. I just didn't want to come then. I was mad because I didn't get an answer. I don't need one now.

LEADER: I think it's an important issue. It's not a question of taking attendance. It has to do with the commitment to the group and to yourself in recovery. If people have a commitment to the group, that's great. Then we can work together. We are not here to set up rules and be police. It's here for people who want to make a commitment to coming, and to gain insight into themselves. If you want that, that's fine, it's here. It's up to you, and not to the group. It's not so great for us if you are going to come and go. Our work is always looking at how we deal with ourselves, feelings, difficulties we have with other people, and dealing with conflict situations. Lately we've had some of those problems right here. It's not so different here than it is outside of group.

MATT: My feeling is that the last two groups have been talking about attendance. If every group is going to be about attendance then I'm not going to make the trip all the way here and miss making 150 dollars.

LEADER: It's up to you. You decided to join this group for your own reasons. Your own suffering brought you here.

MATT: I'd like to hear someone else's thoughts on this.

DAN: I saw a lot of anger on Matt's part about something. I wasn't sure what it was. No one was forcing you to make a decision, Morgan.

MORGAN: I wanted to know where I stood and I didn't get that.

LEO: We gave you an answer last time. What Matt said is what we said. We'd try to work around it.

DAN: I didn't get the sense that anyone was trying to be unreasonable.

LEO: That's all we said and we left it like that. But your not coming last Thursday, that's something else. If you're going to be angry in one sense about not getting any feedback and then you don't come, then I don't know what you mean. You don't want to come and you didn't care. You just said you didn't feel like coming and you didn't want to deal with it.

MORGAN: I remember saying I need an answer.

LEADER: What kind of answer were you looking for?

MORGAN: I feel like I need this lifeline.

AL: I think it worked the right way. You wanted an answer, and I think people instinctively knew better than to give you a yes-or-no answer. You decided you needed this lifeline more than you needed your work project and you made the decision you thought would work best for you, and it was probably the right one. Time will tell of course, but you made the decision based on your own needs, given some input from the group. Instead of having the group decide for you. "Yes, Morgan, you can; no, Morgan, you can't."

MORGAN: I didn't hear half of this. My sense was that if you miss one or two that's too many, and everyone danced around the issue of what we were going to do, and I'd be missing five or six Thursdays.

NORA: You were angry so you heard what you wanted to hear.

MORGAN: I got angry when I didn't get an answer.

DAN: When I get angry I stop listening. All I can do is focus on my anger. I get blocked up with it.

MATT: There are times I don't feel like coming. We can work something out for work, but for a guy not to come just because he doesn't feel like it or is tired or something like that, I don't think that should be acceptable. You were really angry. You lashed out. You were pissed. You said, " I want a fucking answer! Now!!"

LEADER: Morgan, you've had 3–4 absences in the last month, so it's more than going out of town. Something else is going on we haven't talked about.

MORGAN: I've been feeling the pressure for a month and a half, and I haven't talked about it.

LEO: You've got to do something with it, Morgan. It's your question, but it's also a question for us. If we all took on an attitude, "I don't feel like coming," that's kind of like a reversal to, "If you don't want to do what I want to do, then I don't want anything to do with you." I can get into that myself but I'm trying to change that type of behavior. A lot of times you're not going to get the answer you want to hear. You can't play two things. Sooner or later one of them is going to blow up in your face.

MATT: You can see what it does here to the cohesiveness of the group, like Dan said. This attendance thing has disrupted the whole group for two weeks. It affects everyone in the group. You have a negative attitude about us not caring, but I care about you and I get a lot out of you.

DAN: And we miss you when you're not here.

MATT: When the pressures are building up, this is the place you need to talk about it, not at home alone or with some honey. The group can be to your benefit to help you through some tough times. We all have a common bond. If we can work out your situation here now, I may encounter it down the road later on and look back and say, "Morgan did it this way."

LEADER: Well said.

LEO: I wish life were that easy, where somebody could come along and say I need a decision, and get one.

LEADER: All the people here come here for their problem, whatever that is. But then this group becomes the problem. It's funny in a way.

We're here to learn from each other and listen to each other, reflect on ourselves, and see what makes us tick. We didn't get into it except around attendance. We deal with problems and people here the same way as we do outside of the group.

It is worth emphasizing here again how the group and its members can display and play out characterologic problems in maintaining contact and modulating feelings, and at the same time mobilize the courage and strength to face the crises that their problems precipitate. Even Al is able to move beyond his self-centeredness when addressing Morgan's impatience and intolerance of ambiguity. Ultimately the resolution of Morgan's crisis helps the leader and the group to switch back to Al's wish to drop out.

LEADER: With Al I see it a little differently. I don't think it involves which class he is missing—it's more an issue of his relationship to the group. Some of his comments to the group were very devaluing— putting the group down, and not hearing these people speak out to you in a personal, individual way. I think for some reason things have gotten tough for you here, and it wasn't just that school is wonderful and this is awful and dull, and I will dismiss it rather than deal with it. It seems to me the work you have to do here you haven't done yet. People often do that when they get into difficult areas.

AL: Following your presentation there's nothing I can say that wouldn't be denial or rationalization.

MATT: It boils down to priorities. I know as much as I like all you people, I'd rather be out working. Right now I need to be here. I need to learn how to live sober. If I don't lay a good foundation I know where I'm going to end up. You may think your other priorities are more important, but it leads to a fall. When you start saying I'm not an addict, I'm all cured, then you end up back in the hospital, like me, eleven thousand dollars in debt. I fight with it myself. I say then, "What's six months out of my life, a couple hours a week?" When I got high I'd get high for twelve hours a night sitting on the beach. I didn't get anything out of that except debt and shame. I say to myself, "I'm not going to go over there, but I come here, and I need to be here." Otherwise I'll start saying, "Maybe I can use again, and it won't be like the last time." I think (the leader) put it right, it's what you want. You're in or out. I really get a lot more out of going to A.A., but I can get a lot here too, because I can give and get a lot and I enjoy you guys and ladies. Nine times out of ten I bitch and moan about it, then later I'm glad I came. I always have a few laughs at least since I like to laugh and I like to see Morgan smile instead of frown. (*Matt teases Morgan playfully and gives him a hug*).

AL: I guess if it isn't clear, I've already made the decision to quit this group.

RALPH: You're quitting.

AL: Yeah.

RALPH: Quitter.

(*Group laughs*)

AL: So then there's name calling. I suppose you won't give me a ride home tonight.

RALPH: I'll give you a list of drug dealers. (*Group laughs*) I'm only kidding. I wish you the best of luck.

AL: I don't know what to say. I'm not sure what anyone's concern is. Drugs are still a problem. I worry about that every day, and it's a risk. I've been in recovery for a long time, and now it's time to do something else.

LEADER: Have you gotten any sense from here at all of why you used drugs? Maybe this hasn't been helpful to you.

AL: I think I've learned quite a bit about why I used drugs. I don't want to devalue, but I'd be hesitant to say exactly where that information came from.

LEO: We're all in here not really because of drug problems. We really have underlying problems other than drugs. I think that's it. We all have other things going on within us. Maybe opening the door to use later on. To escape again. There are some areas that aren't settled. Then things pile up on us and it's time to run. I can identify with everybody having underlying problems. They don't have to be the same as mine, and that's a common bond, that we all have problems.

AL: The nice thing is you have that bond with everyone in the world, because everyone has problems.

LEADER: That's true, but irrelevant.

MORGAN: What does that mean?

NORA: So go talk to them about your drug problems! (*laughter*)

MATT: Go down to some barroom and talk to some kid about how you just left the Harvard Cocaine Project because your school is more important and see what they say! I totally disagree with what you're saying. I agree with Leo. The difference between the people who can use cocaine socially and those of us who are addicted is that the addicted have problems dealing with reality on life's terms and a lot of issues such as insecurity and not knowing how to handle situations, relations, false pride, and going around wearing a mask thinking they're cool when they're hurting inside. It does go a lot deeper. I just hope you get help.

Here a key shift occurs from a defensive position to one of disclosure and authenticity never shown by Al before. His characteristic imperious attitude and disavowal of need (so common among cocaine addicts) is for awhile replaced by a more honest acknowledgement of feeling vulnerable and frightened. His softening and yielding to the leader and the group's concern also allows him and the group to obtain a more meaningful connection to childhood hurts and fears, and current characteristic ways of self-regard and self-deception.

MORGAN: Tell them what you told me when we were having dinner about your real feelings about the group.

AL: I told Morgan I didn't find the group great. Not the people but the experience. I wasn't receptive to the group experience, and he said, "Why?" like a good therapist.

LEADER: That he is.

AL: Right. And my answer was that one of the biggest things I learned from doing drugs was that a certain kind of vulnerability in myself was exposed that I never experienced before. Maybe sometime way back in childhood, but since then I made sure I was not going to experience that kind of vulnerability again.

NORA: Vulnerable in what sense?

AL: Loss of control. There was something inside me that I couldn't control. Some feeling or desire. I had allowed myself to concede my life to drugs.

LEADER: And it was like that as a boy?

AL: No doubt, but I haven't located that event.

LEADER: Perhaps it's right here now, in this room.

AL: So there was this vulnerability that had been exposed. And it's scary. Part of doing drugs for me is becoming invulnerable. You just close yourself in and nothing can penetrate it. Not even a bullet. When someone gets shot and it doesn't even phase you that's weird. People should be phased when their life becomes unmanageable. But it doesn't for a long time. So I realize I was out of control, that I had lost all sense of proportion. Now all of a sudden it opens a gate, like a little crack in the dam, it bursts open, and I realize this vulnerability has the potential to spread into all areas of my life, especially since I stopped doing drugs.

LEADER: The vulnerability as a kid, and the vulnerability that comes from loss of control on drugs which can be used to cover that vulnerability, like Paul talks of being tender when drug-free and how that is scary to him instead of being tough on drugs. You felt vulnerable before you turned to drugs?

AL: Not that I felt but that I was. I was vulnerable to this personality defect as I've called it before—that people aren't closed systems.

LEADER: That things can get through even to you.

AL: Right, even to me.

LEADER: Do you get anxious at school?

AL: Enormously!

LEADER: So you're human after all.

MORGAN: Tell them the story you told me.

AL: So I'm explaining to Morgan about the group and that I'm not prepared with this newfound vulnerability to let myself be among a group of people that frankly I don't feel all that close to. It's nothing personal. It can be years before you feel really close to somebody. A forced thing never works. So you come here, and everyone is happy and welcomes your input, and that's real. But the level of friendship where you're open and willing to let that vulnerability be has not come for me. I don't feel it. I may be devaluing again.

LEO: We're all at different stages. Being open is being vulnerable. And it's frightening to have to open up.

NORA: I understand what you're saying, and in lot of ways I feel exactly the same as you do, but I've thought about it, and I think it has to do with trust, and in actuality it has nothing to do with us because you're here to do for yourself. No one else can do that for you. Being vulnerable is a healthy thing, if you can be vulnerable in front of people, and I have a hard time doing that too; it shows you've accepted your feelings in being able to be vulnerable. A lot of it is just fear of these and other people.

As with affects in general, the softening of defenses and the admission of vulnerability and fear by Al is contagious, and it gives Nora and others permission to voice similar feelings. Nora enters into the group for the first time since joining, in her case around her conflict of trust and holding back.

MATT: I agree with Nora. I have a tough time trusting people and it takes me a long time. I know in here I can't bullshit people. I'm with the best liars in the world. It is a trust issue for me. Vulnerability is a good emotion because you let your defenses down.

LEADER: But it hurts.

MATT: Al, you try to analyze everything to the max and intellectualize everything. I do it myself but it's easier to see it in other people.

AL: That's not the reason I'm stopping the group, but it's part of it. Maybe if I stuck with it longer I would learn to be more receptive.

MORGAN: Talk to me about the pain.

AL: I don't remember what I said. What I meant is being vulnerable to pain.

NORA: Look, a little bit of color came into his cheeks.

LEADER: What is the pain in here for you?

MORGAN: We're not talking about the pain of bleeding out the eyes, but of anticipation and participation.

AL: In school now I have enormous pain and anxiety. More than ever before in school. I had a final review for a project. At my review I was burned. The worst review I ever had. You finish a project and pin it up on the wall. There are five critics in front of you. Professors and guest critics, and they talk about your work. It is the culmination of your semester's work. I spent six weeks designing a park. They told me I was ignorant, that my project was ignorant. Now I have a tendency to have brutal, harsh reviews. Here they meant ignorant of the basic rules of landscape architecture.

LEADER: You left out the fountain, the benches?

AL: I left out a couple of ponds. Not because I was ignorant but because I wasn't concentrating. They were right. There were a lot of things wrong with the project. But it was really painful, amazingly painful. Because this happens to me continuously. I get burned in my reviews . Usually I get some kind of dialogue going, but in this case they said down the line I was ignorant.

LEADER: I remember when we first met and you spoke then of how you see yourself as always mucking things up, that you would never be successful. I wonder how this relates to that self-view. It sounds like it comes from the same place.

AL: Just the night before my professor was positive about the project, and so I was feeling great, and stayed up all night doing more drawings. The first critic says in his French accent, "Ignorant." (*Group laughs*) You can't say "fuck you" because he was right.

LEO: I've never seen buildings go up in Boston that weren't messed up. I was doing the sheet rock. The architects designed a door that didn't fit. Can you imagine that?

AL: They were right in their criticisms.

MORGAN: How was it for you Al?

AL: I've had reviews like this before. I've been called naive, ignorant, wrong. In this case it was particularly bad. I don't feel ready to finish school. At the end of this year I finish school, and I don't feel now that then I'll be ready to be a landscape architect. I don't know enough.

DAN: Most lawyers coming out of law school don't even know how to find their way to the bathroom, or write a motion.

AL: There is still a point you should have achieved.

MORGAN: Is there a way this school thing relates to the group? Tie it in, Al.

LEADER: Yours was the worst of all the students in your class.

AL: Yes. There were some projects that were really amazing. It hurt.

LEADER: If they called you those names and you didn't hurt I'd be concerned about you.

AL: It hurt more this time than any other time. I was driving home at 10 at night.

LEADER: Exhausted.

GROUP: And depressed.

AL: Exhausted and depressed, and all your friends talk about it, and lots of people looking for a way to show I just might not know what I'm talking about. So a lot of people welcome this kind of attack on me. I put myself on the line so that these projects have to prove that I am right.

LEADER: Your self-esteem is really tied up in this work.

AL: Absolutely. In any case when they are talking about my work they are talking about me. It's all together.

LEADER: They are talking about you as a landscape architect. Not about you as Al.

AL: No, it is a reflection of my qualities as a human being, whether they think so or not.

MATT: Don't you think that sometimes you might have too high an expectation of yourself?

AL: So I'm driving home and I was crying. I never cry. Maybe five times in the last ten years.

LEO: You're not alone.

AL: So here's the vulnerability. I can't take that everywhere. I'm not worried about recovery. Landscape architecture is what really matters. The group is great but I'm not ready to open myself up in here when I have to do it so often in school.

A major shift occurs here for Al from his earlier devaluing position to now valuing the group after being embraced by them, and his acknowledgement that the locus of the conflict is within him, and not in the group's failings.

LEADER: Are the critics here ready for a review of his performance?

AL: I'm putting myself on the line constantly at school. [As he is now in the group for the first time]

LEO: How much time did you put into it?

AL: Six weeks plus 28 years.

LEO: Did you really put six weeks into it?

AL: No, I didn't because I had to come here.

MATT: You're talking about your vulnerability here, and it's ten times worse at school for you. You're faced with this situation and it gets worse, and you think, "I'm a failure." Your expectations are too high, like mine. I always thought everything I did was wrong. That's how I felt all my life. The only thing I felt I could do good was be a drug addict. If the vulnerability is so bad there, then where are you going to go.

AL: Designing a park and public garden is therapeutic.

MORGAN: I think he put the same effort into school that he did here and he got the same amount out of here that he got out of school. The issue I hear running through all of that is "half-assed" attempts. I think the vulnerability issue is the one he has to surmount.

LEADER: Why are you here telling us all this tonight? This is certainly the most real and open you've ever been.

DAN: I think you do us an injustice, too, to presume we're going to be as harsh as your professors.

LEADER: He may not care about our reviews. I wonder how you dealt with it on Friday when you woke up and over the weekend and how you came here tonight and were willing to open up, and talk for real about these things, particularly since you're quitting.

AL: One, I just had this review and it's something to talk about and another thing is I don't feel all that comfortable about leaving. It's scary to leave.

LEADER: You have this view of your recent work that your whole life is wrapped up in it. This is living in an idea of yourself that is a setup for disaster—this notion that you have to be perfect in your acquisition of knowledge, but most of work is getting along with people and learning as you go.

NORA: You don't seem to me like an ignorant person, and if you really gave it your all I can't see you failing at it. In the back of my mind I have this sneaky suspicion that you're setting yourself up for failure subconsciously, and I wondered if you came from a dysfunctional family or if your father was an alcoholic. It seems to me that your basic behavior patterns are messed up.

AL: It would be my pattern not to put much effort into something because of the fear of failure. Usually I'll put a little effort into it, because then when I fail I know I'm going to fail. But in this project I put so much effort.

LEADER: You had a sense of yourself before you ever came to this group as someone who was going to fail in projects.

AL: This semester was different from every other semester. I thought since I wasn't doing drugs, my design will show that; that my optimism regarding life in general would come through in the project. The criticism was bad at the time. It was a short-lived pain. Then I had to go back and evaluate what they said, and say in what ways were they right and wrong. If I don't do well in the next half of the semester I could flunk the course. I have another project that started today. I need to work in the studio with others and talk with them. There's a lot of interaction and dialogue that happens in that studio atmosphere and I've never done that. [As he is doing in the group tonight]

LEADER: Learning from other people in your interactions with them?

AL: Right. Two days a week. [like here] I can't screw around anymore. I'm taking a chance on recovery though.

LEADER: You've raised many important issues tonight, and made a real connection, and captured everyone's interest.

The leader is satisfied here to simply make a supportive and validating comment about Al's making better contact with the group. The group's effectiveness is evident here in helping Al and others identify their relationship problems and the characterological patterns they automatically employ. That is, their patterns of behavior and the distress and suffering that they generate in their lives outside group surface in the group, and become opportunities for self-examination and change. However, this can occur only because the group is a special place that allows and encourages it. The supportive aspects of this group, with its ethos of safety, comfort, and honesty have evolved over months of getting to know and trust each other. The identification and exposure of hurts, fears, and vulnerabilities occured during this meeting because concerns about safety and nurturance have been fostered and reinforced continuously by the leader and the members.

In this meeting the members are sensitive and perceptive in pinpointing core vulnerabilities with relationships and painful feelings. More important, they astutely identify in themselves and each other the self-defeating defenses and character traits they have adopted to protect themselves. In the MDGT group we create opportunities for group members to discover with each other that their psychological protections are often ineffective and the source of personal defeat.

Nora and the group pick up on this theme, and at the same time give Al a supportive and dignified goodbye.

NORA: You know you set yourself up for failure. I wonder what else you could set yourself up for?

MORGAN: No! The dreaded success!

MATT: When I was in the hospital I said I know I'm going to use drugs again, and someone said to me the same thing you said, Nora, to Al: "If you put half as much energy into thinking you can make it as you do into thinking you're a screw-up you'll have no problem in recovery." I know if I want to I can do it. I felt like a failure all my life, that someone is better than me, that I can't pass this, or I can't do that.

NORA: That attitude really kills you. It's like swimming with boots on.

MATT: Al, I have respect for what you're saying, and respect for what you're doing. I hope that things work out for you. I got more out of you tonight than I have since I met you. I wish you nothing but the best, because I think you're a good guy.

LEADER: What did you think about drink or drugs this weekend?

AL: Not only did it cross my mind, but you know how Morgan talked about the naked blonde in the car drinking champagne?

LEADER: You saw her?

AL: I didn't see her but I kind of saw her. I was in my worst possible situation.

RALPH: Some day a couple of years down the road we'll all be in a park looking for a bench to sit on, cursing Al.(*The group laughs playfully, supportive of Al in a way they never have been before*)

AL: My girlfriend was out of town. I had money. I was in the company of drug dealers. I had to go to court with this kid. I was keeping him company. It's not important.

Note here again Al's characteristic tendency to de-value and trivialize his experience and, as the leader surmises, the emotions that are denied. The leader disagrees that "it's not important," and comments accordingly.

LEADER: It sounds important.

AL: I was going home to work all night long, so the combination of money, drugs, Jane out of town and having to work, it was the ultimate position.

LEADER: We're just about done tonight. I'd like to say to you, Al, that you can call it quitting but the door's open and you're welcome to return.

LEO: You can't just leave us hanging. I want to know what your grade is. I'm sure it's going to be a real good grade.

MATT: See, other people have more confidence in you than you do.

AL: I have confidence. I know I can do it.

NORA: I hope you don't stop coming, really. When I first got clean I rationalized everything everybody said to me and it was a real hard long process. I'm clean nine months today. (*Group applauds and cheers*)

NORA: Shut up! (*laughs*) I feel really strong with my sobriety and I feel set, and I don't feel you're set in that way, and I feel you're in a better position than I was. I was next to nothing, and I'm worried for you. (*Group laughs and supports Al*)

LEADER: School aside, nobody gives you reviews. From the little kid who was vulnerable to the little boy whose family kicked him out to private school when he was 14; the kid who was stealing cars when he was 10. That kid. He's still around, and he sees the world in the same painful way in many respects. The door is open for you. You earned a place here tonight.

AL: The chances are then if you leave it open that I will be back.

The group laughs, hugs Al and Nora, who also opened up for the first time.

LEADER: I don't think it needs to be said, but you came here and said you're not close with anyone here and yet you spoke in a profoundly personal way.

Al never returned to the group, quitting after 30 sessions. The other members on the edge of quitting were to continue. Morgan chose the group over a job promotion, and became an increasingly active, supportive, and insightful group member after this session. Nora began to build on her entry into the group made during this meeting, and months later spoke of her sexuality and trauma with the group. This crisis had passed, with the group shifting dramatically from a superficial focus on whether individuals were going to actually leave or stay to the process of thinking decisions through, reflecting on patterns of character, choice, and self-perception, the common ground issue of vulnerability, and to Al as a person speaking of his hurt for the first time.

CHAPTER IX

Nine for One:
Another Crisis

The meeting we review in this chapter demonstrates the progress and potential of a mature group in a more advanced phase. It is similar in structure to Session #41 when Al dropped out, yet here a similar incident is handled in a more confident, easy fashion by the group, and with a more positive outcome than in Al's case. Its resolution leads to common ground themes as well: managing painful affects, seeing oneself as a failure, and completing what one sets out to do. The group in this advanced phase is extremely confronting yet supportive, with the result that Matt gains new insight into himself and makes the decision to continue in the group.

NORA: I'm awful sick of coming three nights a week.

LEADER: (*playfully*) You're always awful sick of something.

NORA: Hey, you work every day, and go to school two nights a week and come here and see what you think. What's that leave you with— shit! (*The group laughingly teases Nora about this*)

LEADER: What else is there in life?

MITCH: You must have had a tough day.

MATT: I got anxiety up the ying-yang! I just had one of those weeks.

LEADER: Leo's girlfriend liked him to be on drugs. He never thought of leaving her until he began getting straight. I wonder if your wife in some crazy way liked you to be on drugs, and now is not totally comfortable with your recovery?

MATT: Yeah, control. When I was high I was just a yes man because I felt so guilty about what I'd done when I was out of the house. Now we have some good arguments, because I say what I feel, and we never did that before. She doesn't like that. Before if she told me to pull over, I'd pull over. If she said "go to the bathroom there," I'd do it.

LEADER: How did you feel about that situation?

MATT: I felt she's the boss and she likes that, and in some insane way in my head that made it alright for me to go out and do what I did.

LEADER: She misses being the boss.

MATT: We have some arguments, and she knows it's a problem.

LEADER: Matt, let's talk about you now. What's up?

MATT: There's going to be changes at work regarding my shift schedule, so I have a decision to make about staying in this group. I don't want to leave my job. I enjoy it, so I have a lot of anxiety about what I'm going to do, and I've gotten a lot of lip from the guys at work about this situation. I have a lot of anxiety about it.

MORGAN: Is it an either–or thing?

MATT: This group only lasts for six months and it's not my primary means of recovery.

This is a group de-valuing comment that needs to be confronted. Furthermore, it raises the issue of Matt's concern about termination which needs to be clarified.

MATT: I just heard about this today. I could be getting all worked up over nothing. I can't continue here if the schedule changes. The union is getting flack about it from other guys.

LEADER: We can't do much about your union, but here you're saying this is not your primary source of recovery.

MATT: No it's not. It's no offense to anyone in here, but I go to five meetings a week, and after this is over that's what I have to go on.

LEADER: What does that mean for you: "primary source of recovery"?

MATT: Getting the most out of my recovery, and I get that at meetings.

LEADER: Something is missing here for you?

MATT: Nothing is missing here. I just get a lot more out of meetings like big book and step meetings. More than I get out of here. I have to think about the future. I'm not cured. I can't say I went to the Harvard Cocaine group and I'm all better now.

LEADER: You're a funny guy in a way, Matt. You're the guy who said, "I'm going to finish this program. I've never finished anything in my life before that counted." Then other times you say, like in the beginning "This group is not for me, then at the end of so many groups over the last few months you say this group was great! fantastic!" I'm confused. You present two sides.

MATT: You're right. I do that sometimes, but I have to think of the future.

LEADER: I don't know about the future, only your life and recovery now. How come it sounds like when Al was here?

MATT: I never tried to put this first in my own head, because it's going to end in six months.

LEO: Are you in or out, halfway in or halfway out? Forget six months from now.

MATT: You have to think of the future don't you?

LEO: There are goals you set, yes, but you can't project six months from now about anything.

MORGAN: That's so true, Leo. When I made my big decision to stay here, I lost a whole hell of a lot at work. I got kicked down to a lesser group, and out of the high-tech group. (*To Matt*) You were very vocal and dogmatic at the time about what's important, and a lot of what you said was instrumental in helping me to make my decision to stay. I could have gone for what was down the line, stayed on this high-visibility team, or was I going to deal with my recovery right now. That's my career. This is my recovery. The balancing act is hard, but a lot of what Leo said just now and what you said then helped me decide what was most important.

MATT: That's why I came here to throw it out, to get some feedback. I haven't made a decision yet. I have to think about it.

MITCH: You say six weeks from now you got to make a decision. Then you give a whole series of reasons why you've already made the decision. You've already decided you weren't going to come here, and now you're rationalizing it to yourself or to us. You said in four weeks I have to decide about this, then you said this is not your number one thing, and have to think of the future and gave a whole bunch of reasons to stop this, so I don't know where you're at.

MATT: Neither do I. That's why I'm here. Today I had a lot of anxiety about what to do. That's been a pattern in my life. When I get anxiety about something, whether I'm making the right or wrong decision. I have to know my recovery is first.

MORGAN: All the reasons you stated puts your recovery second.

The leader keeps articulating Matt's character pattern, in order to focus him and the group on the central, not the peripheral, issues, no matter what the topic at hand.

LEADER: When Al was talking about school it was about the same issues you bring up, that it's more important than this. Yet you have been so much different here than Al. You've reached out to people here in powerful ways, connected with everyone, and helped shape the direction and tone of this group, and have said how much this means to you. Then there's this other part of you that says the group is without value to you, it means nothing. I have to leave here in six months anyway so why get that involved?

MATT: That's why I need to talk about it. I often feel I can't make a rational decision and live with it, like Nora said, I don't have to deal with it right now, but already I get anxiety about it.

LEADER: What sort of decisions that you've made in your life before set you up like this?

MATT: A lot of the decisions I made were the wrong decisions. A lot of the things I've done in my life got screwed up.

MITCH: That's the decision you made yesterday. Today you decided to be in this program. Tomorrow you may decide something else, so the decision you made for today is not irreversible. Is this group worth it? If it's a waste of time, then that's a decision you've got to make for yourself. All that stuff with your union and so on is irrelevant. You make a decision today about being in this group. If you change your mind tomorrow that doesn't mean the decision you made today was wrong. Both of them could be perfectly right, even if they're the opposite decisions. You're making the decision too complicated. You're involving the union, your medical clearance, and all this other stuff that has nothing to do with the decision you've got to make today.

MATT: I can let anxiety get to me.

LEADER: That sounds like an important issue, this anxiety you've mentioned tonight. You said you have a pattern of seeing yourself as not able to deal well with anxiety and making decisions.

MATT: When I heard about it today I felt a lot of anxiety.

LEADER: Who doesn't feel anxiety? But you see yourself as the guy who never finishes anything, who always makes the wrong decisions

MATT: I usually jump to the first decision that comes to mind, and a lot of the time it's the wrong one, instead of slowly thinking it out.

LEADER: Maybe other people here have times they feel something like what you're talking about. Morgan went through this struggle with his job, and Dan, and Leo today was broken down in his truck on Route 9 and felt upset.

MORGAN: At the risk of raising your wrath, man, I got to say I feel I'm being prepared more than anything else, by what you are saying, for an eventuality. I don't feel I'm being asked an opinion, or for the group to help you. I'd like you to respond to that, man.

MATT: That's your opinion (said defensively). That's not right. The decision is mine. What you people think about me is…

MORGAN: Wait! Don't even say it won't make a difference!

MATT: (defensively) I've got to live with my decision. I'm not going to let you or anyone make my decision for me.

Nora helps articulate Matt's character patterns and illustrates the notion of psychological relapse that Matt is playing out as he prepares to jettison the group.

NORA: Think about it like this. Think of all this anxiety you have. Think of how you always reacted when you were full of anxiety, and reverted back to the old behavior, and as soon as you found out this bullshit about your job, what did you do? You reverted right back to this old behavior. That's the decision you've come to. Fuck the program. Fuck this, and that's that, right? With the anxiety you just revert back, because you don't think clearly, and you don't know what you're doing.

LEADER: Is that hard to hear?

MATT: No, she's right. That's why I came here. Anxiety is a very big issue.

LEADER: Let's talk about that, Matt. Managing difficult feelings. People go through many difficult times in life, drugs or no drugs. Six months or six years from now there's always a situation to be faced, a decision to be made, in a program or not. This anxiety sounds like an old thing.

MATT: Fear and anxiety have always been a big issue.

LEADER: Were you anxious about coming here tonight?

MATT: No, because I needed to talk, I need help.

LEADER: Some nights you seem so connected to the group, but tonight you seem so far away, so unconnected.

It seems important for Matt to see himself as one who needs help, who can't cope, who makes mistakes, and quits everything.

MATT: I'm a sick person. You have to understand that. Don't listen to what I say, listen to what I don't say. (*Group laughs*) That's how sick I am.

MITCH: You keep saying the opposite thing. You say to Morgan: "I don't care what you say. I've got to make the decision myself," then the next minute you say, "I need your help."

MATT: Have you ever been confused in your life?

MITCH: Yes! When I get the most anxious I'm on my way to go cop drugs. You revert back to the same behavior. These events are an excuse to do the behavior you maybe want to do, that is the most comfortable for you. Not to use drugs necessarily, but to get rid of this group.

MATT: You've never heard me say, tell me if I'm wrong, that I don't want to come to this group anymore.

LEADER: Matt, you've said it more than anyone in this room, from the first group you attended. You always have two voices about this. One is that this group means very little to me, and is not for me. The other is this group is great , I really like the people in here and get a lot out of being here. You said last week "I'm a runner. I run all the time."

MATT: Maybe I've said something bad about this group on one occasion.

MORGAN: One occasion a night.

MITCH: You said it tonight. That A.A. was for you but not this group.

NORA: You'd better not say that or we'll all kick you. (*Group laughs*)

Their laughter reflects the group's ability to attend to the content of Matt's conflict in a supportive way without being drawn into the sharing of his perception, or without feeling the group is in any real jeopardy of dissolution.

MATT: What I said was this is not my primary source of recovery and it isn't. I'm being honest with you. That's the way it is, and whether you guys disagree or not that's your problem.

LEADER: Matt, what you say now has the quality of devaluing the group.

MATT: I don't mean to hurt anybody's feelings.

LEADER: You tell us the group is not important to you, and other times you say how valuable this group is to you.

Matt, like many group members, tends to see all situations in black-and-white terms. It is difficult to live with ambivalence or uncertainty. His view of the world is one where all is clear and well-defined, where each event is either 100% or 0%, and the middle ground is unbearable.

MATT: Have other people said that too or is it just me?

LEADER: I don't want this to be like it's nine against one. That's not a fair fight. What decision you make is your decision. It reminds me of the night with Al again in so many ways, and I don't want to see you go.

MATT: All this anxiety I have is over nothing.

DAN: The decision you have to make is whether you're going to continue in the group or not.

LEADER: How you deal with your anxiety with the group is more central right now. Could it be that maybe in a way you like this feeling of anxiety, that it's comfortable and predictable, like an old sweater.

MATT: Maybe Nora's right, and Morgan too. Maybe I like that feeling of the worry and the uncertainty, and I can get overwhelmed with things. It does feel comfortable in a way. When this thing came up at work today I thought, "I've got to make a decision right away if I'm going to be in this group or not," and another part of me said, "I don't have to make a decision right now. I don't want to leave this. It is a part of my recovery," and what you said tonight about my being a runner—I'd not thought of that, and I need to hear that.

LEADER: You've always expressed a lot of ambivalence here about the group, but you've stuck with it nonetheless. You said when you began and decided to stay that you were going to finish this, that you've never finished anything in your life, and that this was a goal for you.

The group leader here supportively underscores Matt's inability to tolerate his ambivalence. At the same time he reminds him of his characteristic tendency to convert feelings (in this case, anxiety) into action, namely his characteristic pattern of withdrawal and not completing things.

MATT: That means a lot to me to remember that, and I have a different frame of mind now than when I walked in tonight.

LEADER: I wonder if there were other times in your life when you got excited about something, and thought it was good, and was for you, and was something special, and then after a while you began to lose interest, devalue it, and scrap it?

MATT: A lot of it was when I was younger.

LEADER: Tell us about one of those times.

MATT: I was all psyched for the Boy Scouts, just like here, then I got in and I said it's not for me.

LEADER: How far did you get, what rank?

RALPH: Brownie! (*Group roars with laughter*).

MATT: A lot of the things I joined I did with my brother, Sam. He finished all of them and I never did.

LEADER: What does your family think of you being in this group?

MATT: They think it's good.

LEADER: They could care less?

MATT: I don't know if they could care less. They're not calling me to ask how was the Harvard group. I think a lot of my family has that fear, like my wife does, that I'm going to go back to coke, because that was my pattern before.

LEADER: To quit something and then go back?

MATT: The way they look at it is, like my wife gives me a lot of support but she has a lot of fear of the future, about what's going to happen, what decisions are going to get made, and my family is kind of skeptical because I was in a hospital before.

LEADER: You're going to have to do a lot to convince them. If you quit the group they wouldn't be that surprised?

MATT: Probably not.

LEADER: If you finished it they might be surprised.

MATT: A lot of times in my life I was influenced by what other people thought about me. I want to change that.

MORGAN: He has a good point, Matt. If you finished they'd be seriously surprised. That would be great.

LEADER: Maybe not. Maybe he wouldn't like being in that position of having succeeded at something like this.

PAUL: Your family doesn't even know what happened today, right, so forget what they think. Whether or not you stay in Harvard Cocaine is not the most important issue. That you stay in recovery is the most important issue. Harvard Cocaine is a good productive step toward recovery. You stay because of you, not because your wife is going to feel better that you decided to stay. Big deal, what she thinks. What if you stay in Harvard Cocaine and relapse, what then? You'll have screwed yourself. If you don't want to be someplace, man, you're not going to be there. You only get as much out of this as you put into it. If you sit there every week with an attitude like I don't want to be here, like I did, mind you, for many weeks, and I had to change that attitude. If you sit here with that attitude you're not going to get out of this program what you should. The most important decision is for you to make the decision that's right for you, not for your wife.

LEADER: (*returning to Matt and the underlying themes as the group moves to more peripheral issues*) Is that your older brother you're talking about?

MATT: My younger brother, Sam. We were around the same age. I felt inferior to my brother all my life.

LEADER: How did that work in your family? How did it get to be that way?

MORGAN: So he's the finisher and you're the quitter. So it'd be real easy for you to stay in that old role.

MATT: A lot of what happens in my life and even today, the first thing that comes naturally to me is what I've done all my life. It's like what Nora said, when I get that anxiety and fear what comes natural to me is to run or to quit or to back out and say forget it. When this happened today, the thing that came naturally to me is to say, "I've got to quit this thing." That's what happened, and another part of me said, "You don't have to quit this thing." It was a back and forth thing, and I get overwhelmed. I have a tough time making a decision. I'm confused.

LEADER: Welcome to the earth, Matt.

MORGAN: Me too, man. I know my addictive behaviors really led me down a garden path. One of the things I picked up from N.A. was that stopping drugs is just a little part of it. The greatest part of the battle is changing yourself, and my rule now is to do just the opposite of what my body wants to do. So don't let anyone make it sound like it's easy, man. It's not easy, and with my family, to hell with them. I'm going to show them a different me. If I used to run away and my family expects me to run away, I'm not going to quit. Everyone in here is a damn quitter. My family expects me to be a quitter. I'm going to surprise them this time. I'm not going to quit, and that was a big part of my decision to stay here, and a big part of my recovery.

PAUL: This will do a lot for you man.

MATT: As much as I say I'm confused, that I say one thing and feel another, that's a pattern in my life, and you people help me see that.

LEADER: Hopefully we can speak about it in a friendly way, even though it comes out in warlike tones sometimes. The way we hurt your feelings.

MORGAN: The hot seat returns.

MATT: Even if my feelings got hurt, it doesn't mean I'm going to go use behind it. It's part of growing up.

LEADER: How were your feelings hurt here?

MATT: Like you said, it felt like 9 against 1, and I'm sitting here thinking what the hell is this? Why are they getting on my case?

MORGAN: One night they jumped on me, and one night they jumped on Al, and I didn't think Al was going to come back the next night. Those were the nights we all learned the most.

DAN: Like me when I didn't have a job.

MORGAN: Yeah. Those were the nights we got the most self-awakening. *The first time it happens it feels like it's nine against one, but it's really nine for one, man.*

LEADER: That's nicely said, Morgan.

MATT: I learned that at Stonecliff. After two days being confronted by my peers I wanted to run. I said there's no way I'm going to sit in that room and let twenty guys lay into me. I said "I'm out of here."

MITCH: Let's talk about anxiety a minute because anxiety is something I thrived on. When the coke got really bad and I wasn't getting high anymore and it was just paranoia, what I lived on was what it was like before I did it, because I knew when I did it I'd be sweating and feel awful, but before I'd be anticipating, like how it was for me twenty years ago when it was good. Anxiety always comes when I'm doing something I'm not supposed to be doing, or not doing what I'm supposed to be doing. When I was teaching I'd always put off the grading papers, so part of me wanted to be anxious for some reason, just like you Matt when you said you are comfortable being anxious. I should've been doing my work, and I'd be up late doing coke. I can recognize these feelings now. When I'm sitting in a bar and anxious because I should be somewhere else doing something else. A part of that must have been positive for me to keep doing it all the time. I'd put off things until the last minute, right to the edge.

LEADER: Seeing yourself as "I'm the type of guy who can always get it done at the last minute," and so never does it until the last moment.

MITCH: That I can do this incredible amount of work in this very short time.

LEADER: The other side of this is there's a part of each of us that's like Matt, that has a younger brother that makes us feel we really can't cut it, and we see ourselves deep down in these negative ways, that no matter how hard we try we really can't do it, and it's all somehow a fake, that I'd like to be able to live drug-free or have good relationships or feel good about myself, but it's not really possible, not for me. Even when this thinking is not true in fact. But like Nora said, this way of thinking and feeling comes up immediately at times, and we relapse into the painful, automatic ways we have of seeing ourselves.

LEO: The addiction talks to us like this. I can handle it now, even when I know that's the disease talking shit to me, that I don't have to attend to this anymore or to be attentive to my sickness. As soon as I start to stand up on my own two feet there's this thing that starts, and then you go back to the same old thing.

Leo's insight about the nature of character patterns is as true for self-governance as it is for governance in general—"The price of freedom is eternal vigilance." He instructs us that in a sense the work of group therapy entails an aspect of life that continually involves "unfinished business." Our character patterns, and especially the vulnerabilities they disguise, change very slowly. They automatically drive and govern us, and at times of difficulty, the most problematic and self-defeating aspects of our character structure surface, often beyond our awareness. One of the main values of psychotherapy is that we become more aware of our character patterns and the feelings, relationships, and circumstances that heighten our most self-defeating patterns. To this extent, as treatment expands awareness and as we mature, we take charge of our character patterns rather than our character patterns taking charge of us. Group psychotherapy offers the added advantage of directly observing these patterns unfolding, thereby providing a more immediate chance to observe "psycho- (or character) analysis in action" (Flapan and Fenchel, 1987).

In this case Leo's thoughts also offer Mitch the opportunity to reflect on his own tendency to perpetuate a self-image of failing.

MITCH: I never thought of myself as a quitter. I've finished a lot of things, but a lot of important things I quit on. I never finished my degree and I used to wonder why. I did more work than I needed to but didn't get it done. I never actually bring important things to completion. If you never finished it you can't fail and I'd always think of myself as just kind of a flunkie, a charlatan, a phony, and I was afraid of finishing it off. I don't know what the reasons are. Finishing the most important things I backed off from.

In this instance the group member seems to suggest that it is easier in some respects to be the person with the painful feelings that I invent and control than to be free and suffer the feelings that come with life. (Khantzian 1987a).

LEADER: When I worked long ago in an alcohol detox, a guy once said to me, "I'd like to get well, but not that well." What would it mean not to just live drug-free, but to live as the person who finishes his doctorate, who completes this program, who works his marriage out, who can bear the real pains and pleasures of our lives, to be the person who finishes things, then what, and then you have to come to new terms with life and yourself, because the old excuses are gone. If you break some of those old crippling patterns, like "I'm just Matt, Sam's older brother, I'm a screw-up." If that were just history and not a living part of the present, and it sounds like it is part of the present here, and there's something comfortable about that when you can identify yourself in this narrow way, rather than I'm a guy who finishes things if I want to, I'm a guy who takes care of business, I'm a guy who can deal with and not be destroyed by painful feelings, or the ambivalence of marriage, and other relationships; that none of them are valid reasons to go back and be just the kid who screws up. That psychological relapse and drug relapse are both struggles that have to be dealt with always.

MORGAN: Don't you hate it man when your family keeps you chained back where you were twenty years ago? I have a sister who's the most negative bitch in the world. She holds everyone in the family to the way they were then. My other brother is still the one who steals everyone's candy, and I'm still the one that gets over. These people have changed out of their roles, but she still beats everybody with that old stuff, and I'm tired of it. I'm sure you've got someone in your family like that. Everyone's got one. One day it dawned on me that I am my sister. It's the most depressing thought I ever had, because I do the same shit to me she did to all of us. I'll say to myself, "You always were a big fake," or "You don't really want to push it to the edge and find out because you'll find out you're not much. "

From the initial issue of attendance the group has moved into a rich, complex, deepened reflection on themselves around many of the central MDGT foci: issues of affect tolerance, character style, the effects of the past on current functioning, negative introjects, psychological relapse, and seeing new options for themselves.

PAUL: Matt, let me make a point to you, man. My whole life I made excuses to myself for not completing things. Just like what you are doing now. You can use this situation and make it so you don't complete your goal, which was to complete the program. And even though I did this program half-ass I completed it, man. I see those same tendencies in me. When my mother died I used that as an excuse not to finish high school when I was eight months away from graduating. The same thing all the way down the line for me, man. I should be out of high school now. Go ahead and stick to it and don't make excuses to quit. I stuck to it here. Don't let the bureaucracy of your job affect what you want to do with yourself and your life, man, and to hell with your family. You want to complete the program. You feel like you're a quitter, and this program is a step for you in the right direction. As many times as I wanted to leave and didn't feel I needed it anymore, I stuck in there. It's easier for you to leave than it is for you to stay, so stay. Otherwise you'll regret quitting again. Give it a chance.

The group members do the bulk of the work, rather effortlessly and gracefully reaching out to the member in crisis, drawing on the successful history of the group that has shared many good times and moving moments together. Senior members who are near completion are able to leave a legacy to the newer members who are repeating their own earlier struggles.

Members in these groups begin to see the locus of their problems within themselves, not in the drugs, in other people, or other obsessions. This is a turning point in the life of the group, as they can now begin to use this new learning outside the group in other conflict situations. They display, after a relatively short time in treatment, a capacity for objectivity and reflection, and are able to formulate in a sophisticated way their character patterns, and begin to explore behavioral and psychological options.

This group meeting began in crisis, about to lose one of its key members. It ended favorably as Matt continued and did well in group and ultimately completed treatment. What began as an endangered venture several months ago, with the group on the verge of fragmentation, has led to increased self-awareness, a greater sense of personal flexibility, and a new sense of choice. Psychological relapse occurred in these groups time and time again, but this time it was elucidated and wrestled with within the group, with a different ending than had characterized earlier challenges in the lives of the group members.

The crises did not end in this group. Mitch later was to be the first person who had a drug relapse. Morgan struggled with his drinking and denial. Nora and Morgan one night stormed out of the group in a rage, though they returned and dealt with it next session. Leo, Dan, and Paul completed treatment. There was a celebration, and then the work continued.

The leader continually attempts to refocus the group on the task of MDGT, not on drugs or drug-related behaviors, but on the person. This applies to any other issue or crisis that arises in the group. The leader and the group are always looking at the process, not the content, the character structure, defenses, and capacities for choice, not the drugs or drug-related problems per se. Working through the group crises, the drug relapses and life problems are the road to a cohesive group.

As in the groups above, members drop out, as Al eventually did. Yet even his treatment appeared positive at its end, as he made a more genuine connection with the group. It is the leader's job to do whatever it takes to keep a member in treatment, without sacrificing the integrity and safety of the group, while allowing and respecting members autonomy. The leader walks the line between trying to preserve group membership and being prepared to periodically lose a member. The important outcome sought is not whether the member stays or leaves, i.e. not on the content of the outcome, but on the process, on how the decision was arrived at, not quickly, or heatedly, not what the choice is to be, but how the choice was made. This process of reflection is part of the transmuting process that provides members with a way to look at drug use or impulsive action during moments of crisis in their daily lives when the urge to psychological and drug relapse is strong.

We are all wounded, more or less. The MDGT group, initially attractive to the members for its focus on cocaine, becomes a place of healing for some of the wounds that precipitate or drive drug use. The supportive atmosphere of the group and supportive techniques of the leader are the conditions that allow for the expressive work where the wounded, hidden parts of the self can be made both public and conscious and thus repaired.

CHAPTER X

Nora's Story: The Work of the Advanced Group

Several months have now elapsed since the group was in crisis. Matt and Nora were both about to prematurely terminate. Matt felt that N.A. and A.A. meetings were of more benefit to him than MDGT, and Nora was still angry about being the only woman in a group of eight men. Although she remained in the group, her participation was minimal and her attendance sporadic. The group eventually confronted Nora about her poor attitude and surly expression. Several days later she spoke to the group of her homosexuality for the first time. This secret-telling marked a turning point for Nora and the group. The following transcript picks up the group three weeks after Nora's dramatic disclosure. Her role in group since that time has changed to one of humor, insight, and leadership. Matt, who had always resisted joining in, now emerges as the heart of the group, openly exploring his own problems and reaching out to new and prospective members as they express their own ambivalence and resistance to joining the group.

The MDGT group is based on a six-month, rotating membership model, so in this night's group we have six members, including Nora and Matt, near the end of their treatment, and five members who are just beginning. The presence of the senior members makes this a very different group for the newer members compared to the time when Matt and Nora were beginning. Then there were no senior members who had made it through, no history of crisis, no group tradition, and no method of problem resolution. The group is now simultaneously at the advanced and the beginning phases, shifting back and forth between these phases as the hour progresses.

The role of the leader too is markedly different from the earlier sessions we have described, for now the senior members are able to understand the four core areas of MDGT on their own and model the focus of the work for newer members, bringing them in, and maintaining cohesiveness.

GROUP VIGNETTE #8

The leader in this hour sets the direction of the group in a fortuitously rich way.

LEADER: I was impressed by something Matt said to me after group the other night about Nora, and I was hoping you'd tell Nora and the group about that.

MATT: I was saying that since you've come out and shared with us what was going on in your life a couple of weeks ago, what a change there has been in you here in group. Your whole attitude, your personality, the way you've helped the group, and really become part of the group now and shared has just been unbelievable to me! I was telling my individual counselor earlier tonight that it's been one of the best things that has happened since I've been here. It's just seeing someone here share something that personal, and then seeing the difference in them that is so striking.

NORA: I feel a lot better and much more comfortable in the group. I can share what's really going on with me now and not hold anything back. It's made it a lot more bearable for me. A lot of the time I spent in this group I had a lot of anger because I couldn't get my points across, and I wanted to quit coming. My individual therapist kept encouraging me to share my personal life with all of you. Well, it's been an issue with me all of my life and it's not just a drug-related issue.

Nora has finally made contact with the group around the issue of her sexuality. In an important sense, though, it is not so much the content of the revelation that is significant as it is the process of disclosure, the reaching out to others and making herself vulnerable, and the playing out in the group of a recurrent and familiar relational problem. It is striking that her connection with others leads to a remarkable shift in Nora's personality and functioning in group. Gone are the angry, bristly looks, the toughness, and distance from others. Evident instead is her sense of comfort and enhanced well-being. She is now able to tolerate painful feelings, reveal a depth of herself not shown before, and get the group interested in the common ground theme of how the problems of addiction are often rooted in early problems of basic trust. In addition, for the new members, many of whom have had no prior treatment experiences, she models the process of therapy in both its supportive and expressive aspects. She makes it clear that the thrust of the group's work is not centered on cocaine, but on self, and that it can become in time a safe and salutary place for others to follow her example.

Though Nora has finally come into her own at the very end of the six months by not quitting and becoming a vital member of the group, the dramatic nature and timing of her revelation, her subsequent openness, and the members' unquestioningly enthusiastic acceptance of her conversion and explanation of her previous behavior is in some sense suspect. The group members, both in the group and in their lives as addicts, relish the extraordinary and the dramatic. They are less comfortable with the more ordinary, less dramatic, middle ground. They persist in believing that life without drugs can be painless, fulfilling, exciting, and always happy, with little effort on their part. It is as if the only real problems were that the drugs got out of hand, or that one's sexual preference had been a source of rejection, or that where there was no trust before, it can suddenly, magically, come into full and permanent flower. Both the genuine reaching out to each other and the pseudo-intimacy are obvious in the following:

MATT: As an addict, I think one of the biggest issues we all share is that of trust. You displayed here that you trust us and yourself by making the decision to speak with us about what is most personal for you. It's just amazing! The change in you! I think it's great! And I think it's going to help you down the road. You get to know people, and you get a common bond with those people, and you're able to share those things in confidence, and know that what you say is going to stay here, and know that people are not going to look at you differently because of your personal life.

NORA: It was a big relief to me. Everywhere I go I act as if I have to hide the fact that I am a homosexual. It's a lot of pressure, and it has been for me my whole life.

It is often the case that group members harbor a secret about themselves from childhood and adolescence which they experience as shameful, unable to be shared, and which at the same time they think accounts for their addictions and problems in life. While it is often liberating and healing to reveal this secret at an opportune moment in a safe, therapeutic setting, it can then be disappointing to find that not all life's problems are solved by this revelation.

The leader keeps the focus on the process of Nora's decision to connect and continue with the group, de-emphasizing the dramatic sexual revelation and instead underscoring the radical, delightful, all-encompassing shift in her.

LEADER: What is striking to me is not so much the content of what you told us all about your personal life, but the change in you in this short time. It is not a change in the sense that you are radically different as a person. Not at all. But now in group you have been laughing, warm, bubbly, and you have so much to say to people.

ART: Yeah, you're like human! (*Group laughs*)

Alex has been in the group for less than one month, and is tentative about continuing. He is young, out of work, and from a disadvantaged background. Two nights before, Nora made a connection with Alex when she spoke strongly to him about his drifting, unstructured life. He has decided to return tonight in large part because of her intervention. She has given him hope that there are choices where he had seen none, drawing him into the structure of the group, making him feel important, valued, and capable. It is this supportive process, repeated many times over the life of the group, that is the condition for the possibility of the expressive work as new members make and then deepen their connections with others, just as Nora had recently begun to do.

ALEX: You know I was getting bored in group. I was sick of it. We were getting at the issues, but it was getting boring to me. But last group, you all started getting on my case, and you woke me up! I didn't like to hear it that night, and I was saying to myself, "Damn, I wish they'd shut up and leave me alone"; but hey! I went and got a job. I had no structure to my day. I sat at home all day doing nothing and the day was gone. Now I'm trying to do something more positive, and I feel good again. I think because you [Nora] let us know what was happening with you that now you can talk with us, and get like on my case. I didn't like it , but it did me good. It benefited me. I saw a change in you also that was for the better.

Here we see how Nora acted as a catalyst for Alex both by her own example and her actively reaching out to him. He was unconcerned about her sexual secret, but responded strongly to her "getting on his case" and taking a personal interest in him. This made all the difference in his staying in and joining the group, thereby making a important change in his life, and beginning his own recovery. At this early point in treatment only another group member like Nora, in the potent context of the group, and not the group leader alone, could have effected this turnaround. He was headed out the door, and now he is headed in.

The group returns itself to the central themes Nora raised of secrets, trust, and relationships.

MITCH: When I was at Northridge, they said, "You're only as sick as your secrets." It's not what you're hiding, or that it is necessarily wrong, but it's the way that secret affects you. You have to do a variety of things to keep the secret, and be careful of what you say, and who you say it to. It takes a lot of work to do this. It undermines your confidence and rapport with other people. It's important to keep secrets, but in a place like this group, where you are accepted, it works against your recovery and the group. It's important to be able to talk about the things that are deep, problematic, and troubling.

TOM: It seems like in the last couple of weeks since you told us Nora, that a great burden has been lifted from you in here with us. What you couldn't share with us was reflected in the way you were in the group—angry and isolated. I know that when I first came in here it took a couple of months until I started to feel close to the people here. I felt close to you, but there was something about you that kept me out, that made you know "you don't want to get Nora mad!", or else something is going to fly. It took you a long time to share something with us that's really no big deal.

NORA: No big deal to you!

TOM: With that subject, there is a lot of approval or disapproval in society, and to bring that into a group is hard.

NORA: I was afraid that someone was going to say something in here, and that I would get angry and have to punch him or her in the face, because to me to insult my person and my sexuality would be the worst. I would revert back to old behavior (*laughs*).

LEADER: You must have been disappointed when you didn't get a chance to hit anybody, when the group surprised you.

NORA: Yeah! I was that afraid one of you guys was going to make me angry. I was sure that you'd be insensitive, and then I'd just be humiliated. I was positive of that.

MITCH: What's interesting there is that you took a chance. I don't want to minimize what you shared with us, but it was not that big a deal to us to accept that. We can empathize with the difficulties such a disclosure can cause a person, but the scenarios you attached to this revelation were purely interior for you.

NORA: It's been a problem for me my whole life, and not just in this group. My mother was also a lesbian, and that affected my father and brothers a lot when I was younger. I always felt I had to protect other people's feelings from being hurt because I saw how much it hurt them, and that just carried on my whole life—that I didn't want to hurt anybody's feelings because of my sexuality. But it has made me miserable. I have been protecting people when I didn't have to.

MITCH: You gave Alex some very good advice, and you've been very helpful to a lot of us in the last few weeks, but before I always felt since you were holding back and wouldn't share parts of you your advice was limited. Now, it has more depth of resonance and truth, since you are committed and invested in this group. It's easy to sit back and criticize other people when you're detached. Now those things you say ring more true for me.

NORA: I wasn't detached. I just wasn't saying anything, and got aggravated, because I had this secret and didn't know how to get rid of it, and it really stood in my way here, and I was stuck, and was going to quit the group. I guess I've gotten so good at this over the years it hasn't been a problem for me. I have blocked a lot of people completely out of my life, and this is where it's been a problem.

LEADER: Yet in here, in this group, for some reason, you let us in when you didn't have to, and you stayed when you didn't want to.

NORA: If I had wanted this six months to be useless to me I could have kept up that way, but the guys did encourage me, although they did make me very angry, to discuss this. I have to thank the group for this. I had to make this group work for myself. This was a big problem in my life, and it has been a problem all of my life, and hopefully after this experience here, that is going to change for me.

DIANE: For you, with men, it is that you want to protect their feelings. For me it is fear of rejection. This group is mostly men, and when I told them I was going out with a woman, I thought I'd be rejected.

Diane identifies herself as a lesbian and a bulimic, with a long history of intravenous drug use. Her identity is centered around her addictions, and her social life around various twelve-step groups. She is new to the group, and had told the other members of her sexual preference just after Nora spoke of hers. She was to remain in the group for three months, leave to enter an inpatient center for eating disorders for two months before returning to complete the group. Diane in later groups raises the question of the nature of addiction: is it a "disease" of which one is the helpless victim, requiring medically-based "treatment," or is it a self-medicating flight from oneself and genuine connection with others, the treatment for which is making a connection with herself and others?

MATT: There's a lot more sincerity about you Nora when you talk now. You've become an unbelievable asset to this group. You said what you had to say, and we've seen a change come about in you in such a short time. When I first came around here, I thought six months was an eternity, and I wanted to drop out right away. Now, with only a month left for me, I don't want to leave. I already have some fears about it. I've come so close to the people in this group, and to see changes like that come about in people in recovery, that's what it's all about. It's one thing putting down drugs and drink, but to change...! There's a lot more to it than just not drinking or drugging. I think there's a lot of underlying feelings and reasons why we drank and drugged—the issues in our lives. And to see people face them here, I think that's a major step in staying straight.

TOM: (*to Nora*) I used to sit here and try and figure out why you had such a bad attitude in here. I thought maybe it was work, or something. When you told us, it was such a relief for me. I thought, "OK, that's normal. That explains it."

ART: Nora, you and I came in here at the same time. It was so nice for that to come out, and to be a part of this group when you shared that, instead of the time we wasted talking about attendance and drinking. I really got something out of you letting us in, and I felt for you and admired you for what you did here. Personally, I haven't had a sexual thought in a year. Honest to God. I'm so wrapped up in this recovery thing I just blocked it out. Maybe I have to start thinking about it. And I have no idea what my orientation is going to be.

MITCH: So you have options! (*Group laughs*)

DIANE: It definitely opened the way for me to see you be able to say something like that, and let me follow in your footsteps. That was a horrible night for me when you spoke. I was gritting my teeth, and my stomach was in knots. But it was great for me when you did that.

NORA: I remember the group before that night you all confronted me about my angry attitude. I had to give that a lot of thought, and I knew it was not good and was doing bad things to the group, and it was making it miserable for me. I either had to open up or quit.

MITCH: I learned from that too. We bumped heads, Nora. I don't regret what I said, but I regret the way I said it sometimes. I realized then too how I affect other people, how I cause confrontations that don't need to take place by the way I say things. I regret the way I say things sometimes. I'm not saying I've changed but I've begun to recognize problems I have with people, in the way I talk and respond to people. Sometimes the way I express things is actually counterproductive to what I want to say. That's something I learned here lately.

NORA: You have changed a lot like that, Mitch.

MATT: That's what this group is to me. You have 10–12 people, and everybody becomes a part of the group. You have a lot of different personalities. A lot of people are dealing with different issues, but they have the same underlying cause. And when one person holds back, you hear how it affects the cohesiveness of the group. And it's great that the newcomers here see that too. This will be one of the things that will stand out for me from this whole time. I give you a lot of credit for saying that, since it's a sensitive and personal issue. Now you can look back when you're done and know you got something important out of here, and gave us a great deal, instead of looking back, and thinking that you had wasted six whole months.

LEADER: I remember last fall. Matt almost gone. Nora on her way out the door. Yet you both stayed, and what a difference it has made to the group, and to the new people. You have been vital to the success of this group. It might be hard for the new members to imagine how different Matt and Nora were back then not different as people, but different in their capacity to laugh, speak, and give to others. It was a tough time for both of them for a long time. Attendance was an important issue when the group was struggling. That's where the group was at then, on the edge of breaking up. You stuck in there, and stuck together.

Mitch now makes an important observation about the comings and goings of group members in the short-term rotating membership model we employ. Mitch speaks of living with conflict and ambiguity rather than the glossing over that characterizes Matt's overly optimistic stance.

MITCH: I can see now, Nora, that even though you might not have shared so much with the earlier group, at least you knew them, and that was comfortable. Now we have four new members, and it's hard to keep making that new attachment and commitment to the new group as it changes membership. I get comfortable, then all of a sudden the group changes. It's hard. I was feeling this Tuesday night, with the new members. I said to myself, "This is just too much, I'm having a hard time dealing with this."

MATT: That's what it's all about. When one door closes, another one opens. I like to see new people coming in here, as hard as it is, since I have trouble letting a newcomer get close. I'm sure it's just as hard for the newcomers, or harder. They feel like they're outcasts, and want to become a part of the group, and wonder when they will be like us. We've all been there. It just takes time.

Jeff is a man in his late thirties who used heroin and cocaine intravenously for over twenty years. His story is that of a superb athlete who was headed for the pros before he got heavily involved in drugs in college and wasted his talents. He lives to this day with the pain of this loss sustained in his early twenties, a loss very similar in nature to that of several other group members.

JEFF (brand new member): I sit here trying to follow what is happening. Myself, I have a problem with trust. I gave a big part of me before and I got burned. I have a problem with letting down my shield. I listened to what Nora said about giving that revelation about her personal life which was a major step for her, but we're all here and we have one common bond. We're all addicts, and we're trying to get our lives together. I think we're spending too much time on her being gay or whatever, and we're drifting away from the purpose we are here for.

Jeff speaks of his relationship problems, and then quickly runs from them, wanting to more narrowly focus the group on the idea that drug use is the only problem shared and the only one worth discussing. Nora then strongly counters with her view that addiction is only the meeting ground and the starting point for a recovery grounded in self-esteem reparation, enhanced self-care, a greater ability to tolerate painful feelings, and increased insight into core relationship conflicts, leading hopefully to a more accepting and realistic sense of self and others. Nora understands that the common bond is not addiction by itself, but the dysphoria and suffering that addiction seeks to allay.

NORA: This group isn't actually for dealing with drugs in general as it is for dealing with life's issues that may be causing you to return to a drug. If you can't work something out within a group of people you feel close to then how are you going to survive with people you don't feel so close to in the outside world? How are you going to deal with your pressures on the outside if you can't deal with them in here with people who do share a common bond? That's what this group is all about! It's to learn things about yourself and to try and understand your feelings so that when you do go out there and are having troubles, you've learned here how to deal with that situation, and how to begin to let down some of those barriers that keep people out, and begin to let people in. That's an addict's main problem. They just want to put up that wall and don't want to let anybody in, and can't accept anything from anybody, and just do drugs instead. This group does have a good purpose, and it doesn't always seem to be drug-related *but a lot of issues in life aren't drug-related that do cause people to have drug-related problems.*

LEADER: That's sure well said. I wish I could say it half as well.

ALEX: It's like she said. It's not just to deal with the drug itself. For me it was easy in a way to put down the coke. What I'm dealing with now is hard! I don't think I could have made it this far without this group, to be honest.

LEADER: Alex! Are you alright?!

ALEX: I put myself in dangerous situations a lot. And I don't know why. Last week you told me I was setting myself up to use again by not working, and blaming my girlfriend, and getting impatient. I did the same thing the last time I went back and used.

DIANE: It's familiar though. It's easier, even though it hurts. The feelings I'm going through now are a lot harder to deal with. I was watching a tv show the other night about a guy whose father was dying of cancer. I sat there and cried, and I haven't done that or faced my father's dying in a long time. What I normally would do would be to pick something up, whether it be drugs or food or alcohol or sex to escape those feelings. Turning to my addictions is more comfortable than the new uncomfortable feeling of facing pain and confusion without drugs.

LEADER: We're going to stop in a minute. I'd like to go back to Jeff. What you had to say is very important. What this group is about is talking about the issue of trust, for example, you just mentioned. That might have a lot to do with what is going on in your life. That is part of your pattern, your character, the way you see the world. For Nora, it was in that same ballpark, and she did something in here that was remarkable. It wasn't whether she was gay or not, and she didn't even have to do this, but for her own reasons, she decided to speak with us, to use this group to talk about what she viewed as important to her. And in its wake she is different in the group. The content seems unimportant in a way next to the way she told it, and the way she joined this group at long last. It is as if everyone runs their game and the way they see the world here with each other, and begins to see there might be other ways to see themselves and to do things differently.

TOM: For me this is the best type of therapy I've ever had, because it makes me take a look at myself. Maybe what Nora says has no relevance to myself, but it makes me wonder what's going on with me, and makes me take a look at myself. I always look at this group as my little mock society. I come here and deal with the people and deal with my angers, different problems, and dope-related issues, and it gives me strength to go out and make it so many days without picking up.

Here is testimony to a model of treatment for cocaine addiction for severely chemically-dependent persons that is not focused on drug use, drug-related behaviors, and relapse prevention so much as it is on fostering greater insight into oneself and the healing power of connection with others in a modified psychodynamic group therapy context. The power of this short-term model of treatment for cocaine addiction is that members stay in treatment, enjoy and use the group, have very low rates of relapse while in the group, and often turn their lives around in a short time.

CHAPTER XI

Technique and Technical Issues

In this final chapter on MDGT we offer some guidelines on technique and technical issues. For the better part of this manual we have tried to convey how groups work by generally highlighting certain foci and overriding themes, or in particular, by presenting process material to demonstrate group interaction, development, and progression. In more narrowly focusing on certain issues in this chapter, the guidelines offered are intended to be neither exhaustive nor definitive. They are offered more in the nature of suggestions and examples to assist the therapist in anticipating recurrent themes, concerns, and problems that arise in group psychotherapy with substance abusers. Our hope would be that the experience and views reflected in these guidelines will help the practitioner to maintain a healthy balance between the inevitable uncertainties and the exciting possibilities that our group members present to us as therapists as they attempt to work out their substance abuse and life problems with each other in group therapy.

THE REQUIREMENT OF INDIVIDUAL
COUNSELING OR THERAPY

The reasons people, especially substance abusers, need groups, are often the same reasons that keep them out of groups. Substance abusers are avoidant, counterdependent, and self-absorbed. Groups are powerful antidotes to these characteristics but members need special individual psychotherapeutic help to overcome their resistances and avail themselves of the corrective experiences groups can provide.

Working with addicts's problems of distress, self-contempt, loneliness, and dependency, the empathic clinician is often able to understand why they have chosen a drug–alcohol "solution." Yet, even as they yield in recovery from their drug solution and abstain, it becomes evident that the substances and the vulnerabilities they mask are only part of their problem. What is more formidable and in greater need of modification are the range of characteristic defenses and traits that addicts adopt to disguise or deny their suffering or being lost. Instead of revealing or admitting to difficulty, they more often posture with attitudes of self-sufficiency and disavowal of need and act as if they can solve life problems on their own, if they can admit they have them at all.

To place individuals in groups without lending individual therapeutic guidance, especially at first, can be extraordinarily threatening and bewildering. For addicts it is even more formidable. Given their intolerance of distress and contact and the isolation and distrust that their concerns engender, we should not be surprised that asking such individuals to join a group and rely on and expose themselves to others may seem heroic if not futile. Their often profound counterdependence and deeper layers of shame make it unlikely that they will accept the care and help of others or will reveal their more engageable human qualities.

In our experience we have been impressed with how important an individual counseling or therapeutic relationship can be in brokering and holding substance abusers to the experience of joining and becoming a member of a psychotherapeutic group. As we have discussed elsewhere (Khantzian, 1985b, 1986), the active, supportive, and empathic roles that an individual therapeutic relationship provides can be powerfully alliance building and assist addicts in facing many aspects of life that have otherwise seemed undoable without drugs. This relationship can also be employed in the service of enlisting addicts to accept the beneficial experiences of group psychotherapy. Fears, prejudices, shame, and resistances about groups can be identified, voiced, and explored. When the individual treatment relationship overlaps with and/or parallels the group experience, the therapist and patient are afforded a unique opportunity to monitor and focus on the sources of difficulties of being in group, which might not soon enough or effectively enough be addressed to avoid premature dropouts.

Our experience suggests that for the most part a flexible arrangement is possible when deciding whether the group and individual therapists should be the same or different, the duration of simultaneous individual and group therapy, the possiblity of involvement with self-help groups, and the ongoing focus of the individual versus the group therapy. There are advantages and disadvantages when the group therapist is the same as the individual therapist. When the therapist is the same for both the group and individual treatment, however, he/she is often better positioned to evaluate patient needs and receptivity in both contexts and judge which symptomatic and characterologic problems are better dealt with in individual therapy, and which are better dealt with in group (Khantzian, 1988).

ABSTINENCE AND RELAPSE

Achieving and maintaining abstinence from substances is an ongoing process. Although many group members surprise us and themselves almost immediately about its achievability, in many instances, and especially at first, the craving or desire to use substances by many others remains a major challenge and source of difficulty. In fact, much of the success of self-help groups such as A.A. and N.A. rests on their ability, literally in a "step"-wise fashion, to help individuals establish abstinence by focussing on their inability to control the use of substances and to acknowledge that they are addicts or alcoholics (Brown, 1985). By espousing a "disease" concept of alcoholism and addiction, self-help groups place emphasis on the substance as the "necessary and sufficient" causative agent, and thus insist on absolute control, namely abstinence, as the only way to arrest the disease process or illness. Although at first glance a self-medication hypothesis of addictive disorders, which this manual in part subsumes, might seem at odds with a disease concept, we do not believe operationally or clinically that these formulations or approaches are incompatible or need compete. Dodes (1988), for one, has eloquently articulated how and why a psychodynamic approach can be effectively combined with self-help groups.

As we have spelled out in this manual, self-regulation problems involving affects, self-esteem, relationships and self-care are at the root of addictive disorders, and the use of substances is a symptom of these vulnerabilities. At the same time they are an attempt to "cure" the vulnerabilities. Such a perspective necessarily requires the clinician to understand that for many the use of substances and/or the felt need for them is a symptom that does not go away easily. The substances have become an important part of the addict's or alcoholic's psychological organization, often as an important coping mechanism. On this basis, addicts' dread of abstinence is understandable. Nevertheless, it must also be acknowledged that it is a symptom that can kill. In this respect alcoholism and addiction must often be treated as a condition that cannot wait on an understanding of root causes. This has become dramatically evident with cocaine dependence in which the progression of the addictive process with all its attendant risks of morbidity and mortality is often measured over weeks or months (e.g. compared to the more often indolent, but just as devastating, course of alcoholism which more often spans two to three decades).

The challenge in group psychotherapy is to harness and integrate the uncompromising insistence of self-help groups on control (i.e abstinence) with the best of clinical traditions which place a premium on empathy and understanding as the pathway toward a more permanent and long-lasting recovery. The group leader in this respect, as in so many other respects, has a major responsibility for demonstrating, modelling, and evoking responses among the members which address the emergent and symptomatic aspects of relapse. There is a need for the leader as well as the members to balance the requirement for abstinence with a measure of forbearance and understanding when the inevitable lapses and relapses occur. In some instances this might require that the leader and members focus on and explore the subtleties of an affect state or a blow to one's self-esteem that caused a relatively benign isolated use of drugs for one of the members. Or the challenge might be to harness the passion and power of group concern and influence when another member requires major confrontation, such as when a relapse is unrelenting and life threatening. In the latter instance, the best outcome might be for the group leader and members to have the member in jeopardy accept more intensive help such as hospitalization. Moreover, in our approach, we have tried to indicate that as much as abstinence involves a process, we believe that relapse involves a process as well. The actual reversion to resuming drug/alcohol use is usually evident psychologically far in advance of the act of using. In this respect we view relapse as a process that involves psychological factors and vulnerabilities. Accordingly, we cultivate among the members the need to alert themselves and each other to pre-drug use, symptomatic behaviors, and characterological telltales that might forewarn or herald relapse to the actual use of substances.

The Structure of the Group—Safety, Comfort, and Stability

For any therapeutic group to function effectively constant consideration must be given to factors of safety, comfort, and stability. This is especially so for substance abuse groups, given the major difficulties addicts have experienced with the dangers, dis-ease, and instability involved in drug–alcohol adaptations. To structure and maintain these conditions requires that the leader pay special attention to the composition of the group, how people listen to and talk with each other, how to deal with disruptive-destructive behaviors (inside and outside group), and the specific and general factors which assure group cohesiveness. Beyond the factors of confidentiality, consistency, and support stressed throughout this manual, which are the mainstays for safety, comfort, and stability, we expand further here on several other considerations that we believe are important.

Most group therapists would agree that the composition of a group—the number and characteristics of its members—is an important determinant of a group's viability and effectiveness. Groups for substance abusers are no exception. In our experience we have found that eight to ten members works best. Such a number permits a more natural unfolding, interaction, and progression, without placing an unnecessary burden on the leader or on any one member (as is often the case when only three or four members are present) to speak or provide the needed responses. It also makes it more manageable and comfortable for those who need or prefer to listen and to be more passive until they are ready to speak, and yet for those who speak and actively interact more readily and are able to focus on their own needs, this size group forces them to be more conscious and responsive to the needs of others. Furthermore, when a reaction of understanding, empathy, or validation occurs from members in response to a particular member in crisis or distress, it is strikingly more effective and meaningful when it is spontaneous and forthcoming form a group of eight to ten members, compared to how a similar response can feel forced or begged in a smaller group. This becomes even more apparent and important at times of group attrition when old members are leaving and they have not yet been replaced by new members. Furthermore, as we have indicated, because MDGT rests on the assumption that what is therapeutic or corrective does not rest with the leader alone, the number of members is particularly important in determining the possibilities for the imaginative, unforced, and insightful responses necessary for understanding self and others in group.

In addition to the number of members in group, characteristics of the members, including issues of severity of dysfunction, balance, and matching, are important. Generally (but there are exceptions), severely immobilized and/or suicidally depressed members do not do well in group because they heighten the group's and their own sense of inefficacy. Similarly, severely disorganized or threatening individuals can demoralize or retard group morale and effectiveness. Yet invariably, to some degree these problems emerge in the history of a group and the members, and especially the leader, are forced to play more active, intervening, limit setting, and modulating roles to contain or offset the effects of disturbed or disturbing members. For example, the group leader might need to actively draw out or speak for a very depressed, withdrawn member, even at the the risk of striking out. In doing so, the leader gives voice to his or her and the member's sense of helplessness, in order to demonstrate that the other members are neither alone with nor responsible for the despair such members engender. In other instances, for example with a verbally aggressive or abusive member, the leader might need to intervene to draw the anger to him/herself in order to counter the disorganizing and destructive effect on the member(s) and the group as a whole if it goes unchecked.

Finally, as we believe the process material in this manual demonstrates, individuals are remarkably sensible and sensitive when they gather in groups to help each other. To this extent, it is reasonable to assume there are at least as many forces at work in a group to assure cohesion and growth as there are forces that threaten fragmentation and regression. The group therapist in assuming the mantle of leadership can operate to co-opt and harness these positive elements and forestall the negative ones. In his or her manner of listening and speaking he can demonstrate, evoke, facilitate, and produce responses that contain or discourage fragmentation and reinforce those that result in group cohesion. Especially early in a group's history, the leader must be evocative, active, and if necessary forceful, to create the proper climate for safety, comfort, and stability. Woodward and McGrath (1988), in this respect, have legitimately argued that the leader might even function charismatically (i.e. by authoritative, helpful, and giving) to meet patient needs, especially early in treatment. Subsequently, the leader and the members can trust that, properly led and maintained, the group will progress and grow in providing the responses that are needed to maintain abstinence, recovery, and individual maturation.

SELF-DISCLOSURE AND BEING REAL

It is difficult to practice pretend or pretense in groups. This is as true for the leader as it is for the members. In this section we deal with the ways the leader responds when his feelings and behavior are questioned, how group leaders should respond to questions directed to them about their personal lives, and whether they should generally be reserved or open in their style. Freud's dictum to be oneself is still a useful guide. Nevertheless, the need (and we believe the necessity) to be genuine must also be balanced against the need to not excessively burden the work of the group by disclosures and responses that cause excessive focus on the leader and his/her issues. In this respect it is our opinion that the leader should practice what we have preached elsewhere in this manual, namely to strive for a "middle-ground."

Part of the balance the leader strikes between disclosure and reserve should be guided by the balance MDGT attempts to achieve between the supportive and expressive aspects of the work. On the supportive side we encourage authentic concern and responsiveness for the real achievements, distress, and problems the members experience or endure; on the expressive side we allow enough ambiguity and detachment to help the members play out with and identify in each other the character flaws that govern or perpetuate their dilemmas. To this extent questions or issues directed to or focused on the leader might be part of a genuine need to know or to identify with the leader or part of the often warm and friendly interplay characteristic of MDGT. At other times it might represent a resistance and the playing out of a member's character defects by making the leader an external target of their internal and interpersonal difficulties. Some questions and issues directed to leaders are so loaded in their nature or timing (for example, has the leader used cocaine or is he/she recovering?) that an answer would stimulate too much diversion or dissatisfaction. In such instances our experience indicates that it is best to not answer, but to explain the reasons behind the decision, including the leader's discomfort and concerns about how his/her response(s) might deleteriously affect the work and participation of the group as a whole or some of its members. In other instances during light banter, especially as groups are convening or breaking up, members often inquire about family ("Do you have children?"), talk about sports or movies ("Did you see the ballgame—[or]—Dustin Hoffman in …?") or vacations. Most of the time these questions are benign and friendly in nature. In these instances it is our belief that a friendly and honest exchange is advisable, and moreover, to do otherwise would artificially engender and unnecessarily amplify the interaction.

ACTIVITY/PASSIVITY—THE LEADER, THE MEMBERS

We are all more or less burdened and blessed by the way we are in our psychological nature and the way that this nature is expressed in our basic modes of responding to the inner and outer world. Much of this is in the nature of temperament and thus not easily modified. We believe the modes of activity and passivity are particularly important ones upon which to focus and be aware of in relation to group psychotherapy. Whether exercised or expressed without awareness, or unbridled and in the extreme, by either the leader or members, excessive activity or passivity can produce some of the most bedeviling and demoralizing aspects of group work.

The group leader has a particular responsibility to be aware of his/her penchant for activity or passivity and its effect on the group in general and on particular members. Similarly, the leader needs to be aware of how the activity—passivity modes are expressed by the group as a whole (each group develops its own dynamics), and how the extreme activity or passivity of any one member affects that member, other members, and the group. The leader needs to be aware in extreme cases of the need for him/her to play containing, initiating, activating or modulating roles, to model for the group members and to encourage to do the same for each other. Often for the leaders it is useful to reflect about or speak openly of their own tendency for activity (or passivity) and to speculate on how it interferes or helps with the work of the group. At other times the leader might contrast opposite modes in several members to help them appreciate how their modes affect their relationships inside and outside group. In our opinion it is less important whether one is cryptic and passive or expansive and active. Rather, the leader and members must develop a growing awareness as to how they are, and how this affects others and the possibilities, and at times necessity, for modification and change.

COMINGS AND GOINGS

Someone has referred to the departures, absences, disappointments, and changes that occur in relationships as the "little deaths." How we deal with them often forebodes how we deal with life's more threatening and eventualities. Because substance abusers and addicts so frequently court "near death" experiences with their substances and attendant behaviors, we believe there is a basis to speculate that they test or court in the extreme, feelings about life that they are otherwise unable or unwilling to endure in more ordinary ways. Groups can be extraordinarily beneficial in countering these extreme tendencies and helping substance abusers to test out a more middle ground for experiencing and bearing emotions. The comings and goings in the life of the group are particularly important in this respect.

Although absences, tardiness, growth, and attrition in groups can be the stuff of group dysfunction and crisis (as the process material in this manual demonstrates), these developments can also be the basis for the leader and members to explore and work out the range of feelings and reactions they evoke that might otherwise, and characteristically, go unrecognized and/or expressed maladaptively. In our approach, although we place expectations on members' behaviors involving absence and tardiness, for example, our emphasis is more on converting troubling behaviors into opportunities for self-examination, change, and growth. The group leader can be invaluable in helping the members to create a practicing ground for accessing, identifying, and expressing emotions that the group life engenders, especially those involving the inevitable departures, absences, changes, and special relationships that occur. In our experience, however, there is a considerable degree of variability in how these developments are experienced and manifested. The group leader needs to be vigilant in creating an optimum climate that allows a natural unfolding of reactions suited to the unique qualities of the group and the persons involved, while at the same time avoiding the pitfalls of the extreme, namely, to emotionally ignore or overplay how, for example, a member's absence, tardiness, or planned termination affects the members, the leader, and the group as a whole. Once again, we strive for the middle ground and work to circumvent the extremes of paralysis and no reaction at all on the one hand, and inauthenticity and pseudo-emotion on the other.

These principles of responding apply not only to the tardiness, absences, and the departures of group members, but to other developments in the life of the group such as growth, attrition, and extra-group relationships. The reactions of the leader, individual members, and the group as a whole can vary considerably depending on the situation, event, or members involved.

Sometimes, unanticipated or not, a group might suddenly lose, or conversely, gain several members. At such times, sadness or a sense of loss (i.e. for the absent members or the group as it was) might be the dominant affect or theme for some or all of the members; in another case, the group's attention might shift to a theme of enjoying the emergence of untapped leadership qualities in one of the members around the process of group growth or attrition. A word is also in order about extra-group relationships and activities. Although a risk always remains about unfair and divisive pairings or groupings outside the group, in general we believe it is both unnatural and undoable to prohibit them. This is especially so, given the contemporary trends for so much formal and informal contact (often very needed) that occurs among members participating in self-help groups. The leader can neither encourage nor discourage these relationships, but he/she can share concerns and experiences about potential problems and risks, and single out obvious hazards as they develop. The main concern of the group leader and members should be an expressed awareness of the possibility of unfair or divisive groupings, and that the members must remain open and honest about their extra-group relationships and activities. Whatever the changes or developments, their significance should not be condemned or exaggerated. Rather, they should be seen as opportunities to enjoy gains and successes and to bear disappointment and distress in the group, while at the same time linking the group experiences to life events outside group. In this way the group developments impart to the members a growing and deeper appreciation of how similar life events outside group, unrecognized and unprocessed, have precipitated and maintained drug use.

STYLES OF THE LEADERS

Therapeutic technique and style is best guided by our understanding of the origins and nature of the members' vulnerabilities. Our work with substance abusers indicates that most of them have been exposed to extreme environments developmentally, involving traumatic abuse, deprivation, or neglect. As a consequence they suffer from special disabilities and character structures that affect their capacities for self-regulation and relationships. Group therapists as much as, if not more than, individual therapists must keep these considerations in mind in the way they conduct themselves and their treatment of substance abusers. For the most part, then, and understandably, substance abusers do not respond well to the traditions of therapeutic passivity, the blank screen, or the uncovering techniques derived from psychoanalysis of the neuroses (Khantzian, 1986). Instead they need therapists who can actively and empathically help to engage them and each other around their vulnerabilities and the self-defeating defenses and behaviors they adopt to avoid their distress and suffering.

In general, MDGT allows for a range of qualities and styles in the leader. As we indicated, however, extremes in modes of behavior or style on the part of the therapist as well as members, especially ones of extreme passivity and unresponsivness, are counterproductive if not antitherapeutic. A friendly, unpretentious and reasonably open manner, within the constraints of one's usual makeup or temperament, will serve the therapist and group best. As circumstances and group and individual needs dictate, the therapist should be flexible enough to fill and model a range of roles, one moment prepared to be firm and directive if the group founders or a member behaves offensively; at another time prepared to yield when, for example, the group members need feedback and modification if they excessively focus on a particular issue or person.

The main allies for therapeutic practice, nevertheless, remain the listening and observing modes. The involved group therapist is constantly challenged to empathically fine tune to whatever is said at the same time he/she scans for how what transpires affects the other members. Furthermore, as much as there are central concerns in our roles as therapists for carefully taking in, absorbing, and integrating what our group members say and reveal (or disguise) in the group transactions, clearly there are ways and ranges of responding to group members that should also concern us. A strict and narrow focus on resistances and transference, for example, in our opinion, will not work. More often the responsive therapist will find him/herself facilitating and evoking when sensitive problems or painful affect are skirted or avoided. He/she might label and instruct when a member or the group cannot access or identify an emotion or issue, yet, at another time a simple statement of clarification might be sufficient. It is not unusual in our approach for the group leader to seize a moment of crisis or breakthrough to reflect out loud about a person or an issue. The leader in these instances may demonstrate, evoke, or guide members in cultivating a capacity to integrate thoughts and feelings about life situations in the service of forestalling impulses and cultivating in its place more self-reflection, restraint, and circumspection. More rarely, but nevertheless effective and necessary to reach more refractory members, active measures such as coaching, guided focusing, or confrontation on an issue might assist members to grasp or understand a situation that otherwise escapes them.

THE SUPPORTIVE METHOD

Throughout this manual we have stressed that MDGT occurs within a supportive, friendly context. This develops through the members' and leader's active responses of respect, admiration, empathy, and real concern for distress. The leaders in MDGT take special measures to enlist the members as collaborators with them in self-exploration and under-standing. There is a shared responsibility in the group for establishing and maintaining the conditions of safety, comfort, and stability, which are the essential underpinnings of the work. The leader constantly models and demonstrates how respect, curiosity, empathy, undivid-ed/attentive listening, and tactful/careful speaking foster these ends. The members and leaders repeatedly reinforce and encourage these responses. The group discourages pretend and pretense, and in their place fosters honest self-examination and authentic self-expression. The guidelines and reflections we have presented in this final chapter are offered not as rigid precepts or practices. They are offered more to convey a philosophy and attitude about group work with addicts and how the leaders and members can function to best accomplish the task of being helpful to each other.

REFERENCES

Abraham, K. (1908). The psychological relation between sexuality and alcoholism. In Abraham, K. (1960). *Selected papers of Karl Abraham*. New York: Basic Books.

Alonso, A. (1989). *Character change in group therapy*. Grand Rounds presented at The Cambridge Hospital, Cambridge, MA.

Anderson, S. C. (1983). Group therapy with alcoholic clients: A review. *International Journal of the Addictions, 14*, 437–43.

Baker, H. S., & Baker, M. N. (1987). Heinz Kohut's self psychology: An overview. *American Journal of Psychiatry, 144*, 1–9.

Balint, E. (1972). Fair shares and mutual concerns. *International Journal of Psychoanalysis, 53*, 61–65.

Bauer, G. P., & Kobos, J. C. (1984). Short-term psychodynamic psychotherapy: Reflections on the past and current practice. *Psychotherapy, 21* (2), 153–169.

Bean, M. (1984). Clinical implications of models for recovery from alcoholism. In H. J. Shaffer & B. Stimmel (Eds.), *The addictive behaviors*. New York: Haworth Press.

Bernard, H. S., & Klein, R. H. (1977). Some perspectives on time-limited group psychotherapy. *Comprehensive Psychiatry, 18* (6), 579–585.

Bibring, E. (1954). Psychoanalysis and the dynamic therapies. *Journal of the American Psychoanalytic Association, 2*, 745–770.

Blatt, S. J., Berman, W., Bloom-Feschback, S., Sugarman, A., Wilber, C., & Kleber, H. (1984). Psychological assessment of psychopathology in opiate addiction. *Journal of Nervous and Mental Disease, 172*, 156–165.

Blume, S. (1985). Group psychotherapy in the treatment of alcoholism. In S. Zimberg, J. Wallace, & S. B. Blume (Eds.), *Practical approaches to alcoholism psychotherapy* (2d ed.). New York: Plenum.

Borriello, J. F. (1979). Group psychotherapy with acting-out patients: Specific problems and technique. *American Journal of Psychotherapy, 33* (4), 521–530.

Brown, S. (1985). *Treating the alcoholic: A developmental model of recovery*. New York: Wiley.

Brown, S., & Yalom, I. D. (1977). Interactional group therapy with alcoholics. *Journal of Studies on Alcohol, 38* (3), 426–456.

Budman, S. H., & Gurman, A. S. (1988). *The theory and practice of brief therapy*. New York: Guilford Press.

Budman, S., Soldz, S., Demby, A., Feldstein, M., Springer, T., & Davis, M. S. (1989). Cohesion, alliance and outcome in group psychotherapy. *Psychiatry, 52*, 339–350.

Cartwright, A. (1987). Group work with substance abusers: Basic issues and future research. *British Journal of Addiction, 82*, 951–953.

Cooper, D. E. (1987). The role of group psychotherapy in the treatment of substance abusers. *American Journal of Psychotherapy, 41* (1), 55–67.

Crowley, R.(1939). Psychoanalytic literature of drug addiction and alcoholism. *Psychoanalytic Review, 26*, 39–54.

Davanloo, H. (1978). Evaluation criteria for selection of patients for short-term dynamic psychotherapy: A metapsychological approach. In H. Davanloo (Ed.), *Basic principles and techniques in short-term dynamic psychotherapy*. New York: Spectrum.

Deykin, E. Y., Levy, J. D., & Wells, V. (1987). Adolescent depression, alcohol and drug abuse. *American Journal of Public Health, 77*, 178–182.

Dodes, L. (1988). The psychology of combining dynamic psychotherapy and alcoholics anonymous. *Bulletin of the Menninger Clinic, 52*, 283–293.

Dodes, L., & Khantzian, E. (in press). Psychotherapy of substance abusers. In R. Shader, & D. Ciraullo (Eds.), *Clinical manual of chemical dependence*. American Psychiatric Association Press.

Donovan, J. (1986). An etiologic model of alcoholism. *American Journal of Psychiatry, 143*(1), 1–11.

Fenchel, G. H., & Flapan, D. (1985). Resistance in group psychotherapy. *Group, 9* (2), 35–47.

Flapan, D., & Fenchel, G. H. (1987). *The developing ego and the emerging self in group psychotherapy*. Northvale, NJ: Jason Aronson.

Fenichel, O. (1945). *The psychoanalytic theory of neurosis*. New York: W.W. Norton.

Flores, P. J. (1988). *Group psychotherapy with addicted populations*. New York: The Haworth Press.

Freud, S. (1930). *Civilization and its discontents*. New York: W.W. Norton. (1964).

Freud, S. (1905). *Three essays on the theory of sexuality*. London: Standard Edition, 7 (1949).

Fried, E. (1985). The process of change in group psychotherapy. *Group, 9* (3), 3–13.

Fried, E., & Fried, J. A. (1980). Acceptance: A key factor in the treatment of narcissism. In L. R. Wolberg & M. L. Aronson (Eds.), *Group and family therapy 1980*. New York: Brunner/Mazel.

Gawin, F. H., & Kleber, H. D. (1986). Abstinence symptomatology and psychiatric diagnosis in cocaine abusers. *Archives of General Psychiatry, 43*, 107–113.

Gawin, F. H., & Kleber, H. D. (1984). Cocaine abuse treatment. *Archives of General Psychiatry, 41* (903–908).

Gerard, D. L., & Kornetsky, C. (1954). Adolescent opiate addiction: A case study. *Psychiatric Quarterly, 28*, 367–380.

Gerard, D. L., & Kornetsky, C. (1955). Adolescent opiate addiction: A study of control and addict subjects. *Psychiatric Quarterly, 29*, 457–486.

Glover, E. (1932). On the aetiology of drug addiction. In Glover, E. (1956) Selected papers of psychoanalysis. Vol. I: *On the early development of mind*. New York: International Universities Press.

Goldberg, A. (1978). *The psychology of the self*. New York: International Universities Press. Goldberg, D. A., Schuyler, W. R., Bransfield, D., & Savino, P. (1983). Focal group psychotherapy: A dynamic approach. *International Journal of Group Psychotherapy, 33* (4), 413–431.

Gruen, W. (1977). The stages in the development of a therapy group: Tell-tale symptoms and their origin in the dynamic group forces. *Group, 1* (1), 11–25.

Grunebaum, H., & Solomon, L. (1980). Toward a peer theory of group psychotherapy, I: On the developmental significance of peers and play. *International Journal of Group Psychotherapy, 30*, 1, 23–49.

Grunebaum, H., & Solomon, L. (1982). Toward a theory of peer relationships, II: On the stages of social development and their relationship to group psychotherapy. *International Journal of Group Psychotherapy, 32* (3), 283–307.

Grunebaum, H., & Solomon, L. (1987). Peer relationships, self–esteem, and the self. *International Journal of Group Psychotherapy, 37* (4), 475–514.

Gustafson, J. P. (1986). *The complex secret of brief psychotherapy.* New York: W.W. Norton.

Gustafson, J. P. (1984). An integration of brief dynamic psychotherapy. *American Journal of Psychiatry, 141* (8), 935–944.

Guttmacher, J. A. (1973). The concept of character, character problems, and group therapy. *Comprehensive Psychiatry, 14* (6), 513–522.

Guttmacher, J. A., & Birk, L. (1971). Group therapy: What specific therapeutic advantages? *Comprehensive Psychiatry, 12* (6), 546–556.

Homans, G. (1950). *The human group.* New York: Harcourt, Brace, and World.

Kandel, D. B. (1980). Developmental stages in adolescent drug involvement. In D. J. Lettieri, M. Sayers, & H. W. Wallenstein (Eds.), *Theories of Addiction.* NIDA Research Monograph No. 30. DHHS Publication No. ADM 80-967. Washington, D.C.: Superintendent of Documents, U.S. Government Printing Office.

Kaplan, H. I., & Sadock, B. J., (Eds.) (1971). *Comprehensive group psychotherapy.* Baltimore: Williams and Wilkins.

Kaufman, E., & Reoux, J. (1988). Guidelines for the successful psychotherapy of substance abusers. *American Journal of Drug and Alcohol Abuse, 14* (2), 199–209.

Kernberg, O.F. (1983). Psychoanalytic studies of group processes: Theory and applications. In L. Grinspoon (Ed.), *Psychiatry Update, 2*, 21–36. Washington, D.C.: American Psychiatric Press.

Kernberg, O. F. (1986). *Severe personality disorders.* New Haven: Yale University Press.

Khantzian, E. J. (1974a). Opiate addiction: A critique of theory and some implications for treatment. *American Journal of Psychiatry, 28*, 59–70.

Khantzian, E. J. (1974b). Heroin use as an attempt to cope: Clinical observations. *American Journal of Psychiatry, 131*, 160–164.

Khantzian, E. J. (1975). Self-selection and progression in drug dependence. *Psychiatry Digest, 10*, 19–22.

Khantzian, E. J. (1978). The ego, the self and opiate addiction: Theoretical and treatment considerations. *International Review of Psychoanalysis, 5*, 189–198.

Khantzian, E. J. (1979). Impulse problems in addiction: Cause and effect relationships. In H. Wishnie (Ed.), *Working with the impulsive person.* New York: Plenum.

Khantzian, E. J. (1980). An ego-self theory of substance dependence. In D. J. Lettieri, M. Sayers, & H. W. Wallenstein (Eds.), *Theories of addiction*. NIDA Research Monograph No. 30. DHHS Publication No. ADM 80-967. Washington, D.C.: Superintendent of Documents, U.S. Government Printing Office.

Khantzian, E. J. (1981). Some treatment implications of the ego and self disturbances in alcoholism. In M. H. Bean & N.E. Zinberg (Eds.), *Dynamic approaches to the understanding and treatment of alcoholism*. New York: The Free Press.

Khantzian, E. J. (1982). Psychological (structural) vulnerabilities and the specific appeal of narcotics. *Annals of the New York Academy of Sciences, 398*, 24–32.

Khantzian, E. J. (1983). An extreme case of cocaine dependence and marked improvement with methylphenidate treatment. *American Journal of Psychiatry, 140* (6), 484–485.

Khantzian, E. J. (1985a). The self-medication hypothesis of addictive disorders: Focus on heroin and cocaine dependence. *American Journal of Psychiatry, 142* (11), 1259–1264.

Khantzian, E. J. (1985b). Psychotherapeutic interventions with substance abusers—the clinical context. *Journal of Substance Abuse Treatment, 2*, 83–88.

Khantzian, E. J. (1986). A contemporary psychodynamic approach to drug abuse treatment. *American Journal of Drug and Alcohol Abuse, 12* (3), 213–222.

Khantzian, E. J. (1987a). A clinical perspective of the cause–consequence controversy in alcohol and addictive suffering. *Journal of the American Academy of Psychoanalysis, 15* (4), 521–537.

Khantzian, E. J. (1987b). Psychiatric and psychodynamic factors in cocaine dependence. In A. Washton & M. S. Gold (Eds.), *Cocaine*. New York: Guilford Press.

Khantzian, E. J. (1988). The primary care therapist and patient needs in substance abuse treatment. *American Journal of Drug and Alcohol Abuse, 14* (2), 159–167.

Khantzian, E. J., Gawin, F., & Kleber, H. D. (1984). Methylphenidate treatment of cocaine dependence—A preliminary report. *Journal of Substance Abuse Treatment, 1*, 107–112.

Khantzian, E. J., Halliday, K., Golden, S., & McAuliffe, W. (1989). *Group therapy for substance abusers: A psychodynamic approach to relapse prevention*. Paper presented at the National Institute on Drug Abuse Symposium. Atlanta, GA.

Khantzian, E. J., & Khantzian, N. (1984). Cocaine addiction: Is there a psychological predisposition? *Psychiatric Annals, 14* (10), 753–759.

Khantzian, E. J., & Mack, J. E. (1983). Self-preservation and the care of the self-ego instincts reconsidered. In *Psychoanalytic Study of the Child, 38*, 209–232.

Khantzian, E. J., & Mack, J. E. (1989). Alcoholics anonymous and contemporary psychodynamic theory. In Marc Galanter (Ed.), *Recent developments in alcoholism, 7*. New York: Plenum.

Khantzian, E. K., Mack, J. E., & Schatzberg, F. (1974). Heroin use as an attempt to cope: Clinical observations. *American Journal of Psychiatry, 131*, 160–164.

Khantzian, E. J., & Shaffer, H. J. (1981). A contemporary psychoanalytic view of addiction theory and treatment. In J. Lowenstein & P. Ruiz (Eds.). *Substance abuse in the United States: Problems and perspectives*. Baltimore: Williams and Wilkins.

Khantzian, E. J., & Treece, K. (1977). Psychodynamics of drug dependence: An overview. In J. D. Blaine & D. A. Julius (Eds.), *Psychodynamics of drug dependence*. NIDA Research Monograph No. 12; DHEW Publication No. ADM 77-470. Washington, D.C.: Superintendent of Documents, U.S. Government Printing Office.

Khantzian, E. J., & Treece, C. (1985). DSM-III psychiatric diagnosis of narcotic addicts: Recent findings. *Archives of General Psychiatry, 42*, 1067–1071.

Klein, D. F. (1975). Psychopharmacology and the borderline patient. In *Borderline states in psychiatry*. New York: Grune and Stratton.

Klein, R. (1985). Some principles of short-term group therapy. *International Journal of Group Psychotherapy, 35* (3), 309–330.

Knight, R. (1972). The psychodynamics of chronic alcoholism. In S. Miller (Ed.), *Clinician and therapist: The collected papers of Robert P. Knight*. New York: Basic Books. Kohut, H. (1971). *The analysis of the self: A systematic approach to the psychoanalytic treatment of narcissistic personality disorders*. New York: International Universities Press.

Kohut, H. (1977). Preface. In J.D. Blaine & D.A. Julius (Eds.), *Psychodynamics of drug dependence*: NIDA Research Monograph No. 12; DHEW Publication No. ADM 77-470. Washington, D.C.: Superintendent of Documents, U.S. Government Printing Office.

Kosten, T. R., Rounsaville, B. J., & Kleber, H. D. (1987). A 2.5 year follow-up of cocaine use among treated opioid addicts. *Archives of General Psychiatry, 44*, 281–285.

Krystal, H. (1982). Alexythymia and the effectiveness of psychoanalytic treatment. *International Journal of Psychoanalytic Psychotherapy, 9*, 353–388.

Krystal, H., & Raskin, H. A. (1970). *Drug dependence: Aspects of ego function*. Detroit: Wayne State University Press.

Levy, M. (1987). A change in orientation: Therapeutic strategies for the treatment of alcoholism. *Psychotherapy, 24* (4), 786–793.

Luborsky, L. (1984). *Principles of psychoanalytic psychotherapy: A manual for supportive–expressive treatment*. New York: Basic Books.

Luborsky, L., & Crits-Cristoph, P. (1989). A relationship pattern measure: The core conflictual relationship theme. *Psychiatry, 52* (3), 250–259.

Luborsky, L., Woody, G. E., Hole, A., & Velleco, A. (1977). *A treatment manual for supportive–expressive psychoanalytically oriented psychotherapy: Special adaptation for treatment of drug dependence*. (Unpublished manual, 4th ed., 1981).

Mack, J. E. (1981). Alcoholism, a.a., and the governance of the self. In M. Bean & N. E. Zinberg (Eds.), *Dynamic approaches to the understanding and treatment of alcoholism*. New York: Free Press.

Malan, D. H. (1976). *The frontier of brief psychotherapy*. New York: Plenum.

McAuliffe, W. E. (1984). Nontherapeutic opiate addiction in health professionals: A new form of impairment. *American Journal of Drug and Alcohol Abuse, 10* (1), 1–22.

McAuliffe, W. E., & Albert, J. (1990). *The outpatient cocaine cessation group.* Unpublished manuscript.

McAuliffe, W. E., & Ch'ien, J. M..N. (1986). Recovery training and self help: A relapse prevention program for treated opiate addicts. *Journal of Substance Abuse Treatment, 3,* 9–20.

McAuliffe, W. E., Santangelo, S., Magnunson, E., Sobol, A., Rohman, M., & Weissman, J. Risk factors of drug impairment in random samples of physicians and medical students. *International Journal of the Addictions, 9,* 825–841.

McDougall, J. (1984). The "dis-affected" patient: Reflection on affect pathology. *Psychoanalytic Quarterly, 53,* 386–409.

McLellan, A.T., Woody, G., & O'Brien, C. P. (1979). Development of psychiatric illness in drug abusers. *New England Journal of Medicine, 201,* 1310–1314.

Meissner, W. W. (1986). *Psychotherapy and the paranoid process.* New York: Jason Aronson.

Milkman, H., & Frosch, W. A. (1973). On the preferential abuse of heroin and amphetamine. *Journal of Nervous and Mental Disease, 156,* 242–248.

Poey, K. (1985). Guidelines for the practice of brief, dynamic group therapy. *International Journal of Group Psychotherapy, 35* (3), 331–354.

Rado, S. (1933). The psychoanalysis of pharmacothymia. In H. Shaffer & M. E. Burglass (Eds.). *Classic contributions in the addictions* (1981). New York: Brunner/Mazel.

Rosecan, J. S., & Nunes, E. V. (1987). Pharmacological management of cocaine abuse. In H. I. Spitz, & J. S. Rosecan (Eds.), *Cocaine abuse: New directions in treatment and research.* New York: Brunner/Mazel.

Rounsaville, B. J., Gawin, F., & Kleber, H. (1985). Interpersonal psychotherapy adapted for ambulatory cocaine abusers. *American Journal of Drug and Alcohol Abuse, 11* (3&4), 171–191.

Rounsaville, B. J., & Kleber, H. (1985). Psychotherapy/counseling for opiate addicts: Strategies for use in different treatment settings. *International Journal of the Addictions, 20* (6&7), 869–896.

Rounsaville, B. J., Weissman, M. M., Crits-Christoph, K., Wilber, C., & Kleber, H. D. (1982a). Diagnosis and symptoms of depression in opiate addicts: Course and relationship to treatment outcome. *Archives of General Psychiatry, 39,* 151–156.

Rounsaville, B. J., Weissman, M. M., Kleber, H. D., & Wilber, C. (1982b). Heterogeneity of psychiatric diagnosis in treated opiate addicts. *Archives of General Psychiatry, 39,* 161–166.

Sands, P. M., Hanson, P. G., & Sheldon, R. B. (1967). Recurring themes in group psychotherapy with alcoholics. *Psychiatric Quarterly, 41,* 474–482.

Sashin, J. I. *The relationship between fantasy and the ability to feel affect.* Unpublished paper presented at Grand Rounds, The Cambridge Hospital, Cambridge, MA, November 5, 1986.

Schiffer, F. (1988). Psychotherapy of nine successfully treated cocaine abusers: Techniques and dynamics. *Journal of Substance Abuse Treatment, 5,* 131–137.

Sifneos, P. E. (1979). *Short-term dynamic psychotherapy.* New York: Plenum.

Sifneos, P., Apfel-Savitz, R., & Frank, F. (1977). The phenomenon of "alexithymia". *Psychotherapy Psychosomatics, 28,* 47–57.

Spitz, H. I. (1987). Cocaine abuse: Therapeutic group approaches. In H. I. Spitz & J. S. Rosecan (Eds.), *Cocaine abuse.* New York: Brunner/Mazel.

Stone, W., & Gustafson, J. P. (1982). Technique in group psychotherapy of narcissistic and borderline patients. *International Journal of Group Psychotherapy, 32* (1), 29–47.

Treece, C., & Khantzian, E. J. (1986). Psychodynamic factors in the development of drug dependence. *Psychiatric Clinics of North America, 9* (3), 399–412.

Vannicelli, M. (1982). Group psychotherapy with alcoholics. *Journal of Studies on Alcohol, 43* (1), 17–37.

Vannicelli, M. (1988). Group therapy aftercare for alcoholic patients. *International Journal of Group Psychotherapy, 38* (3), 337–353.

Vannicelli, M. (1989). *Group psychotherapy with adult children of alcoholics.* New York: Guilford Press.

Vereby, K. E. (1982). Opioids in mental illness: Theories, clinical observations, and treatment possibilities. *Annals of the New York Academy of Sciences, 398.*

Wallerstein, R. (1986). *Forty-two lives in treatment.* New York: Guilford Press.

Washton, A., & Gold, M. E. (1987). *Cocaine.* New York: Guilford Press.

Weiss, R. D., & Mirin, S. M. (1984). Drug, host and environmental factors in the development of chronic cocaine abuse. In S. M. Mirin (Ed.), *Substance abuse and psychotherapy.* Washington, D.C.: American Psychiatric Press.

Weiss, R. D., & Mirin, S. M. (1986). Subtypes of cocaine abusers. *Psychiatric Clinics of North America, 9,* 491–501.

Weiss, R. D., Mirin, S. M., Griffin, M. L., & Michaels, J. K. (1988). Psychopathology in cocaine abusers: Changing trends. *Journal of Nervous and Mental Diseases, 176* (12), 719–725.

Weiss, R. D., Pope, H. G., & Mirin, S. M. (1985). Treatment of chronic cocaine abuse and attention deficit disorder, residual type with magnesium pemoline. *Drug and Alcohol Dependence, 15,* 69–72.

Weissman, M. M., Slobetz, F., Prusoff, B., Mezritz, M., & Howard, P. (1976). Clinical depression among narcotic addicts maintained on methadone in the community. *American Journal of Psychiatry, 133,* 1434–1438.

Wieder, H., & Kaplan, E. H. (1969). Drug use in adolescents: Psychodynamic meaning and and pharmacogenic effect. In *Psychoanalytic Study of the Child., 24,* 399–431.

Wolberg, L. R. (1967). The technic of short-term psychotherapy. In L. R. Wolberg (Ed.), *Short-term psychotherapy.* New York: Grune and Stratton.

Wolf, A. (1971). Psychoanalysis in groups. In H. I. Kaplan & B. J. Sadock (Eds.), *Comprehensive group psychotherapy.* Baltimore: Williams and Wilkins.

Woodward, B., & McGrath, M. (1988). Charisma in group therapy with recovering substance abusers. *International Journal of Group Psychotherapy, 38* (2), 223–236.

Woody, G. (1977). Psychiatric aspects of opiate dependence: Diagnostic and therapeutic research issues. In J. D. Blaine & D. A. Julius (Eds.), *Psychodynamics of drug dependence.* NIDA Research Monograph No. 12; DHEW Publication No. ADM 77-470. Washington, D.C.: Superintendent of Documents, U.S. Government Printing Office.

Woody, G. E., McLellan, A. T., Luborsky, L., & O'Brien, C. P. (1986). Psychotherapy for substance abuse. In S. M. Mirin (Ed.), *The Psychiatric Clinics of North America, 9,* 547–562.

Wurmser, L. (1974). Psychoanalytic considerations of the etiology of compulsive drug use. *Journal of the American Psychoanalytic Association, 22,* 820–843.

Wurmser, L. (1978). *The hidden dimension: Psychodynamics in compulsive drug use.* New York: Jason Aronson.

Yalom, I. D. (1974). Group psychotherapy and alcoholism. *Annals of New York Academy of Sciences, 233,* 85–103.

Yalom, I. (1985). *The theory and practice of group psychotherapy (3rd ed.).* New York: Basic Books.

Yalom, I. D., Bloch, S., Bond, G., Zimmerman, E., & Qualls, B. (1978). Alcoholics in interactional group therapy. *Archives of General Psychiatry, 35,* 419–425.

Zackon, F., McAuliffe, W. E., & Ch'ien, J. M..N. (1985). *Addict aftercare: Recovery training and self help.* DHHS Publication No. ADM 85-1341. Washington, D.C.: Superintendent of Documents, U.S. Government Printing Office.

Zweben, J. (1987). Recovery-oriented psychotherapy: Facilitating the use of 12-step programs. *Psychotherapy, 19* (3), 243–251.

INDEX

Absence/tardiness, 159–160, *see also* Group therapy, attendance of
Abstinence, 2, 3, 23, 28
  maintaining, 5, 154
  relapse from, 154–156
  strengthening, 28
Acceptance, in group therapy, 20, 80, 85
Acting out behavior, 26, 28
  in antisocial personality disorder, 39
Activity, *see also* Hyperactivity
  preoccupation with, 72, 76
  as quality of group leader, 159–160
  and self-esteem, 10
  in therapeutic process, 4
Addictive personality, 37
Affective disorders; *see also* Feelings
  bipolar type, 31, 36, 41
  in cocaine addiction, 9–10, 31
Affects; *see* Feelings
Aggression, 13, 34–35
Alcohol, as sedative-hypnotic, 35
Alcoholics Anonymous (A.A.), 2, 6, 68, 73–74, 154
Alcoholism, 13, 34, 155
  and defenses, 35
  group work, in, 6, 7; *see also* Alcoholics Anonymous
  modified therapy for, 27
  and self-care vulnerability, 42
Alexithymia, 11, 37, 72
Alonso, A., 24
Ambivalence, intolerance of, 95, 112, 130, 131
Anergia, 9, 10, 35, 38
Anger, 110–111
Antidepressant medication, 38
Antisocial personality disorder, 31, 38, 39
Anxiety, 34, 125, 128, 129, 131, 135

concerning group therapy, 56, 80
  signal, 42
Attention deficit disorder, 36
Autonomy, 85

Bean, M., 27
Bibring, E., 94
Bipolar-type affective disorder, 31, 36, 41
Birk, L., 24
Blaming, 63, 64
Borderline personality disorder, 39
  in cocaine addiction, 31
  in group therapy, 26
Borriello, J.F., 26, 76
Brown, S., 7, 25, 27, 154
Budman, S.H., 25

Cartwright, A., 26
Change, 61, 64, 147
Character structure, 2, 3, 21, 28, 72
  in cocaine addiction, 10
  defenses of, 72–75, 153
  disturbance of, 3, 9
  patterns of, 23, 67–68, 98, 99, 121, 136
  treatment of, 3, 23–24
Charisma, 158
Cocaine, 3, 31–32, 35–43, 84, 114, 155
  affective stability, 3, 9–10
  cognitive disruption in, 3
  as coping mechanism, 32
  in countering depression, 35, 38
  defenses in, 19, 73
  dependency needs in, 40
  disdainful style in, 73, 74
  group therapy for, 25–26
  and narcissistic personality, 19, 31–39, 40
  predisposition for, 36, 37